MW01482365

Copyright © 2015 by Elizabeth Popish.

All rights reserved. No part of this publication may be reproduced, distributed, or transmitted in any form or by any means, including photocopying, recording, digital scanning, or other electronic or mechanical methods, without the prior written permission of the publisher, except in the case of brief quotations embodied in critical reviews and certain other noncommercial uses permitted by copyright law.

For permission requests, please address Elevate Publishing

Editorial Content: AnnaMarie McHargue

Cover Design: Bobby Kuber

Interior Layout: Sarah Smitka

This book may be purchased in bulk for educational, business, organizational or promotional use.

For more information, please email info@elevatepub.com.

Published by Elevate, a division of Elevate Publishing, Boise, ID

ISBN-13: 9781937498825

Library of Congress Control Number: 2015946854

Expanded Joy

52 Projects to Increase the Purpose,
Passion, and Playfulness in Your Life

Elizabeth Popish

Table of Contents

To Steven, Lauren, and Julia
No other joy compares

Introduction

In September 2008, I found myself in a mall bookstore on a mission to find a book. Not a specific book so much as a *type* of book. As a person who had read her way through virtually every phase of life, I was certain the book existed if only I could find it. Unfortunately, I was at a loss to adequately describe the book though more than one employee addressed me, eager to be of assistance. Still, I was convinced I would know it when I saw it.

I wandered, unaided, through the aisles, plucking books at will from the shelves. By the time I had finished I held no fewer than seven books: a compact book of yoga poses, an intellectual's devotional, a glossy entertaining book, a world history book, a gardening book, a lighthearted missive on happiness, and the latest trend in healthy eating. Even cumulatively, the books did not satisfy what I envisioned. With scarcely contained frustration, I returned the books, drove home, and decided to create the book I was unable to find. I began *Expanded Joy*.

At forty-nine, I had one daughter in college out-of-state, another finishing high school, and a husband winding down on a career in veterinary medicine. My own career in educational administration had slowed years earlier to allow more time at home with our girls. As a result, I had been blessed with the freedom to try a number of different ventures, a gift of indulgence that was never lost on me. I delved into interior design for a period, joined three friends in a seasonal garden and home décor store, tried my hand at creative writing, sat on the board of the art museum, received certification in a positive psychology course from a Harvard professor, and took up cross country skiing.

And then, at the cusp of fifty, I stalled. Like an engine that goes from smoothly revving one moment to sputtering the next, I rather abruptly hit a wall — physically, emotionally, mentally, and spiritually. For the first time in my life, I was unsure of what I was meant to do. I simultaneously became restless and lethargic, hypersensitive and unmotivated. I went through the motions of my life on autopilot, doing the things I needed to do, but finding little pleasure in the effort. My family tiptoed around me, aware something wasn't quite right, but unsure of how to help.

It was for this reason that I found myself in the bookstore that day, looking for the book that would map out a new course for me. A book that would restore my equilibrium in the way books had seen me through job interviews and childbirth and running a school and parenting. When my exhaustive search for the book that would magically get me back on track proved fruitless, I understood with a sense of dismay, I would have to create it myself. Though the task felt herculean in scope, I simply could see no other alternative. And so, following Anne Lamott's invaluable advice in *Bird By Bird*, I began to take the task apart, one step at a time.

To begin, I asked myself what it was I was hoping the end result to be. That proved to be the easy part: I wanted to feel joyful again. And not only did I want to feel more joyful, but I wanted to be able to access that joy regardless of what was going on around me. To possess a means for elevating my joy that was independent of my environment. In other words, I wanted to master my own life. To live optimally of my own accord. After brainstorming general areas of optimal living, I eventually settled on seven categories: energetic health, authentic happiness, mental engagement, stress reduction, social connections, creative expression, and altruism. An eighth area of spirituality was intentionally omitted due to a personal belief that churches exist for precisely that purpose.

For three years I worked on the program, becoming as knowledgeable as possible within the various areas. Once I determined the seven categories, I set about developing individual subjects to include in each category and from there, specific implementation strategies. It was not enough to simply *comprehend* a particular theory or concept; I wanted to ensure that my behavior would change as a result of that knowledge. I set up the strategies on a daily, weekly, and monthly schedule, dedicating time each day to the task of joyful living.

When asked by friends how I was spending my time, I would sometimes reference the project, and their responses were both surprising and vindicating. Almost to the person, they were able to empathize with my journey. They, too, had experienced the same malaise I had experienced while they marched steadily toward middle age, though not always in the exact same manner. Nearly all expressed a similar desire to increase the joy in their lives and would often ask if I might share my strategies. In this way, working on the project and visiting with other women about the topic, I began to experience a deepening sense of joy more profound than any I could have imagined.

In 2011, we made a retirement move to Boise, Idaho, and *Expanded Joy* was temporarily shelved. Although I was more invested than ever in what I had learned over the previous three years, I also was certain I would find a comparable class in this moderately large city. Once we were settled, I began combing the area for women's classes in the area of joy and optimal living, obsessively searching opportunities online. But, once again, I came up empty handed. I returned to tweaking my material, working my program, and making acquaintances in our new home.

In 2014, at the urging of a couple friends, I launched my first *Expanded Joy* class to a group of twenty-five women. It resulted in one of the most gratifying experiences of my life. The outpouring of positive response was unlike anything I could have anticipated, and I forever will be grateful and touched by this initial group of dynamic women who gave me the opportunity to share the material in this program. Thanks to their enthusiasm, I had the courage to move forward with this book and the opportunity to influence others in a positive way. This has been proven to be, the ultimate joy.

All strategies within this book are research-based with a preponderance of data proving their effectiveness by leaders in the various fields. They were designed for individual use or with others in a group setting, in much the same way as a book club. If you choose to go the route of a group, each individual strategy could be studied and explored by members of the group before reporting back at a monthly get together. This would allow you not only to work your way through the strategies systematically, but to benefit from the social connection as well – a powerful antidote to premature aging. The impact of other women's comments, humor, experiences, suggestions, and imaginings cannot be overstated. If you are at all inclined, I would urge you to form your own *Expanded Joy* circle with a group of friends, neighbors, acquaintances at church, or work colleagues.

InJOY!
Elizabeth Popish

ACTIVITY SUBJECT AREAS:

These seven themes of optimal living form the foundation of the Expanded Joy program. Each of the fifty-two projects included within this book falls within one of these primary areas.

 + EMOTIONS *(Authentic Happiness)*

Raise your happiness level by increasing the occurrence of positive emotions through the science of happiness

 + ENERGY *(Health and Wellness)*

Discover the critical areas of physical well being to maximize your energy potential

 + ENGAGEMENT *(Intellectual Stimulation)*

Study the upside of meaningful engagement and the powerful concept of "flow"

 + EASE *(Intentional Calm)*

Deflect daily stress with strategies designed to promote genuine serenity and well-being

 + ENCOUNTERS *(Social Connections)*

Celebrate the power of friendship, the perfect antidote for successful aging

 + EXPRESSION *(Creativity)*

Learn why creativity, inherently present in each of us, is an important component of quality living

 + EARTH *(Greater Good)*

Uncover ways to positively impact your community, the nation, and our planet

WHAT MAKES ME HAPPY?

The foolish man seeks happiness in the distance, the wise grows it under his feet.

— JAMES OPPENHEIM

Background

Check any nonfiction book list and you are certain to find titles like *The Happiness Project* and *The Art of Racing in the Rain* devoted to the ubiquitous pursuit of happiness. Long before such books existed, however, a young Englishwoman named Marion Milner was on her own introspective journey toward the discovery of personal happiness and self-fulfillment. In 1926, using the pen name Joanna Field, Marion began keeping a daily journal to discover what triggered the feeling of delight in her daily life. *A Life of One's Own*, chronicling that search, was published in 1934. It attracted the attention of such literary heavyweights as W. H. Auden and Steven Spender, and within a short time, a subsequent book of a similar theme was published titled *An Experiment in Leisure*.

Getting Started

This week, you will be asked to follow Ms. Milner's lead by keeping track of those objects, sensory encounters, places, hobbies, and activities that result in an undeniable feeling of satisfaction when you experience them. This might include such things as getting a pedicure, playing tennis, wearing red, having a glass of wine, doing the crossword puzzle from the paper, the smell of gardenias, a call from your child, salsa dancing, the latest installment of Masterpiece Theater, that luxurious hand cream by your bedside, finding a favorite magazine subscription in the mailbox, or any number of other similarly small delights. This list will be used at a later date for a subsequent activity.

Noteworthy

- The specific feeling of pleasure that comes from indulging in a personal luxury is short lived and embodies only a limited aspect of happiness, but it's an important one. Such momentary treasures not only break up our day, but keep it from becoming too dull and burdensome.

- Research shows those skilled at capturing the joy of the present moment, hanging on to positive feelings and appreciating good things, are less likely to experience depression, stress, guilt, and shame.

- It may take you several weeks to complete your list (use additional sheets of paper if necessary). Review it from time to time to determine if there is anything you would like to add or delete.

Directions: As you go about your week, list those things you discover make you particularly happy.

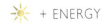

SLEEPING FOR ENERGY

Each night when I go to sleep I die. And the next morning, when I wake up, I am reborn.

— MAHATMA GANDHI

Background

Insomnia is the most common sleep complaint among Americans, and can range from acute (lasting one night to several nights), to chronic (lasting months to years). According to the National Center for Sleep Disorders Research at the National Institutes of Health, some 30–40 percent of adults claim to have symptoms of insomnia within any given year and approximately 10–15 percent claim to suffer from chronic insomnia. Refreshing sleep positively contributes to nearly every aspect of our life including: improved immune system, enhanced memory, increased productivity and performance, and better ability to handle stress. Poor sleep has even been proven to contribute to weight gain as the "good" hormone leptin, which suppresses appetite, is reduced within the body and the "bad" hormone ghrelin, which prompts the body to eat, simultaneously rises.

Getting Started

If you suffer from poor sleep, it may be time to take a look at your sleep hygiene. This refers to certain behaviors you exhibit throughout the day that can positively or negatively affect the quality of your sleep. On the following page you will find a list of sleep hygiene rules that have been proven to make a difference to your snooze time.

Over the course of a week, ascertain which habits you are following and which call for a change in behavior.

Noteworthy

* The five stages of sleep include: Stage 1) a drowsy, relaxed state between waking and sleeping; Stage 2) a light stage of sleep we are easily awakened from; Stages 3 and 4) a deeper, more profound sleep distinguished by very slow delta brainwave patterns; and Stage 5) REM or dream sleep.

* Some individuals, who believe they have insomnia, may actually simply need less sleep than the standard 7–8 hours. If you habitually are not nodding off during sedentary activities or sleeping late on weekends, you simply may be spending more time in bed than you require.

* As we age our sleep quality changes so that we produce less deep sleep and wake more frequently and for longer intervals. By our seventies, deep sleep has all but disappeared.

Directions: Throughout the week, note which of the following sleep hygiene behaviors you are already doing. If you are having difficulty sleeping, take a closer look at those you could alter.

_____ Wake up/go to bed daily within the same 30-minute time frame, even on weekends.

_____ Get 30–60 minutes exercise throughout the day (_insomniacs are typically more sedentary than those without sleep issues_).

_____ Check to see whether prescribed medications may be causing insomnia.

_____ Use your bed for sleep and sex only; office work and electronics need to be done elsewhere (_30 minutes or so of reading to get sleepy is acceptable_).

_____ Stop intake of caffeine after midday, including less obvious sources of caffeine like chocolate, coffee/chocolate ice cream, weight loss pills, pain relievers such as Excedrin, and energy water.

_____ Take a power nap of no more than 20–30 minutes (_avoid altogether with chronic insomnia_).

_____ Stop eating within 3–4 hours of bedtime.

_____ Avoid excessive alcohol, which causes awakening later in the night.

_____ Take a warm bath, shower or hot tub prior to bedtime (_not only will this relax your muscles, but temporarily raises your body temperature, promoting sleep as it begins to fall_).

_____ If you need a small snack just before bed, make it a combination of protein and carbohydrates (_i.e. cereal with milk, cheese and crackers, toast with peanut butter_).

_____ Play soothing music, sip chamomile tea, and use lavender scents to help induce sleep.

_____ Make sure your room is dark (_turn clock away from view_) and cool (_warm rooms are particularly disruptive to sound sleep_).

_____ Work to minimize disruptions of spouse/children/pets (_use earplugs and white noise machine if necessary_).

_____ See doctor to address severe snoring issues for yourself or spouse.

_____ Use moderately firm pillow, comfortable bedding, and sleepwear that breathes.

_____ Just prior to drifting off take 20 cleansing breaths to clear the mind.

_____ Sleep in the fetal position (_on side, knees bent at 90° angle_).

_____ Make your _To Do_ list for following day before retiring.

_____ Consider relaxation exercises, biofeedback or Cognitive Behavior Therapy for anxiety issues.

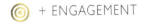

THE BEAUTIFUL BRAIN

I do not feel obliged to believe that the same God who has endowed us with sense, reason, and intellect has intended us to forgo their use.

— GALILEO GALILEI

Background

Thanks to current research in the area of neuroplasticity we now know the brain is constantly reshaping and rewiring itself. The finding that the human brain is actually malleable, rather than unchangeable after a certain age as we once believed, has tremendous ramifications in terms of our role in the ongoing health of our brain. By improving brain function in such areas as alertness and focus, learning and remembering, accuracy, sequencing, speed and fluency, we can go a long way in prolonging or even eliminating age-related neurological diseases like dementia and Alzheimer's. But this does not happen without a concerted effort on our part. A healthy lifestyle in addition to intensive, sustained learning, is essential to enjoying a long and productive life.

Getting Started

It's time to start caring for the brain in the same way we care for the body. One activity that will accomplish both is aerobic exercise. Partaking in regular exercise that gets you winded to the point of gasping for air is not only good for your cardiovascular system, but beneficial to the brain as well. Eating fish, particularly fatty fish such as salmon, is another example of how you can improve cognition. In the coming week, try to incorporate these suggestions along with the tips on the following page into your routine as often as possible.

Noteworthy - Taken from Dr. Merzenich's book *Soft-Wired*

⊙ Unstructured or passive sitting is one of the least productive activities for strengthening the brain. Reduce the amount of time that you are not mentally engaged to some degree. Going about your day with minimal effort or thought involved slowly dulls your brain's capacity.

⊙ Try to find activities that are both demanding and rewarding so that your brain is motivated to engage. For example, the hobby of bird watching requires an intense knowledge of birds including classifications, notable identifying marks, and particular sounds. At the same time the bird enthusiast experiences great satisfaction when spotting a particular species outdoors.

⊙ When practicing new skills and activities, find those that can never be completely mastered. Consciously work to improve both skill and speed. Count each measureable step of progress as success.

Directions: Try to incorporate as many of the following activities into your week as possible. Take notes on strategies tried throughout the week to engage and strengthen the brain.

1. Sign up for a class and participate to the same degree you did as a student. Be a careful listener and focus intently on what is being said. Take notes and try to quiz yourself daily on material.

2. At social gatherings be attentive to names of individuals to whom you are introduced. Repeat their name at some point in the conversation and once home write down as much as you remember about people.

3. Work on jigsaw puzzles in the evening or while watching TV. Work to increase your speed and search for different strategies in locating pieces. Aim for one or two puzzles a month.

4. Ball games such as tennis, softball, or Ping-Pong are particularly good for exercising the brain. Along this line, juggling is a simple activity to engage the brain when you have a few minutes of free time.

5. Play progressive games with a partner, such as chess, that utilize logic.

6. Volunteering and having a defined purpose in life activates the brain in ways those who are more withdrawn from society do not.

7. While walking, pay attention to street names so that you can anticipate their order correctly. Visit a museum and pay close attention to information you encounter. Once you arrive home, try to reconstruct that information in writing.

8. Eat dark chocolate daily, which activates the systems in your brain that pump dopamine, an important brain chemical.

9. Learn a new musical instrument or renew your interest in an abandoned one. Following music uses a different portion of the brain as does studying a foreign language.

10. Consider signing up for an online brain exercise sites, which have been shown to improve brain speed and fluency long after the exercises have been discontinued.

BELLY BREATHING

As long as I am breathing, in my eyes, I am just beginning.

— CRISS JAMI

Background

Deep breathing (called "pranayama" in yoga) dates back more than two thousand years to India where the practice of yoga originated. Meaning "to yoke together" (mind and body), the practice of yoga revolved around the three principles of exercises, breathing, and meditation. Although originally reserved for the religious elite, eventually yoga became more commonplace, spreading to other countries. Today, breathing techniques are still commonly taught in yoga classes, though you don't have to be a yogi to receive the benefits.

Getting Started

Deep, purposeful breathing is perhaps the single most effective tool for combating stress and anxiety, but is often overlooked for the very reason it is so useful — its simplicity. Before committing to daily deep breathing, make sure you are familiar with the correct technique.

Proper Deep Breathing Technique

- *Sit straight in your chair with your spine erect.*
- *Place one hand on your abdominal muscles.*
- *As you inhale, feel your abdomen expand first upward toward your chest.*
- *As you exhale, keep your spine straight, your shoulder blades together and down, and your neck between your shoulders; do not collapse at the heart or mid body.*
- *Your abdomen should contract at the end of the breath cycle*

Noteworthy

- Shallow breathing increases carbon dioxide levels in the blood, causing anxiety, moodiness, muscle atrophy, fatigue, excessive adrenaline, increased heart rate, and high blood pressure. Even "brain fog" is a common side effect of shallow breathing and diminishes with deep breathing. Experts report deep breathing for ten minutes daily can reduce stress levels by as much as 44 percent.

- One way to work deep breathing techniques into your schedule is to practice while sitting in your car at a red light. It may help to place a small sticker in the corner of your mirror to remind yourself to take advantage of spare moments available.

Directions: In the coming week, practice the following breathing exercises until you feel comfortable with them.

Three Breathing Exercises
By Wellness Expert Andrew Weil, M.D.

Bellows Breath (Energy)

- Inhale and exhale rapidly through your nose, keeping your mouth closed but relaxed. Your breaths in and out should be of equal duration, but as short as possible.
- Try for three in and out breath cycles per second. This produces a quick movement of the diaphragm, suggesting a bellows. Breathe normally after each cycle.
- Do not do for more than 15 seconds on your first try. Each time you practice this exercise, you can increase your time by five seconds or so, until you reach a full minute.

4–7–8 Exercise (Relaxation)

- You can do this exercise in any position, but sit with your back straight while learning. Place the tip of your tongue against the ridge of tissue just beyond the upper front teeth, and keep it there the entire exercise. You will be exhaling through your mouth around your tongue; try pursing your lips slightly if this seems awkward.
- Exhale through your mouth completely, making a whooshing sound.
- Close your mouth and inhale quietly through your nose to a mental count of four.
- Hold your breath for a count of seven.
- Exhale completely through your mouth, making a whooshing sound to a count of eight.
- Repeat the cycle three more times for a total of four breaths.

Breath Counting (Meditation)

- Sit in a comfortable position with the spine straight and the head inclined slightly forward. Gently close your eyes and take a few deep breaths. Then let the breath come naturally without trying to influence it. Ideally it will be quiet and slow, but depth and rhythm may vary.
- To begin the exercise, count "one" to yourself as you exhale.
- The next time you exhale, count "two," and so on up to "five."
- Begin a new cycle, counting "one" on the next exhalation.
- Never count higher than "five" and count only when you exhale.
- Try to do this for ten minutes as a form of meditation.

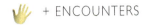

WHO'S IN MY HOUSE?

Shared joy is a double joy, shared sorrow is half a sorrow.

— SWEDISH PROVERB

Background

Research has shown one of the strongest indicators of personal happiness is the depth and breadth of social connections formed throughout our life. It is believed our desire to bond with others originates from an evolutionary need. Humans would not have been able to survive without the help of others, which may be why we strongly resist the break up or dissolution of friendships. Considering two of the major contributors to premature aging are lack of mental stimulation and decreased number of social connections, it pays to make friendship and camaraderie a top priority at all stages of life.

Getting Started

In this exercise you will be asked to take a social connection inventory. Take time to consider thoughtfully all personal relationships, small groups, clubs, and organizations with which you belong or participate. Your list should include individuals that might not live in your city, but with whom you communicate regularly. If you find it difficult to identify even a minimum number of genuine relationships and outside groups, consider setting a personal goal to increase your numbers each year.

Noteworthy

- If you are single rather than married or in a committed relationship, experts recommend having at least ten close friends with whom you share a personal bond.

- Relationships provide us positive feelings, which in turn help attract higher quality relationships, which make you even happier. In this way, you initiate an upward spiral of good fortune when you take the time to invest in relationships.

- People with strong social connections are healthier and tend to live longer than those with few relationships. This may be due to the fact that a key functions of a social bond is the provision of support in time of stress, grief, and trauma.

- If you have difficulty forming new relationships due to a shy nature, consider joining a club, study group, or organization where you can get to know people at your own pace.

Directions: List any and all current relationships and associations in the appropriate space.

1 Who's In My House?
Include your closest friends, family, and confidantes here:

_____   _____

_____   _____

_____   _____

_____   _____

_____   _____

_____   _____

_____   _____

2 Who's In My Neighborhood?
Include close work mates, Bunco groups, spiritual small groups, book clubs, and friends you see regularly here:

_____

_____

_____

_____

_____

_____

3 Who's In My Community?
Include larger organizations, professional cohort groups, work colleagues and friends you see occasionally here:

_____

_____

_____

_____

_____

_____

ADDITIONAL NOTES:

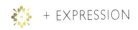

CREATIVE COLLAGE

Imagination is the beginning of creation. You imagine what you desire, you will what you imagine, and at last, you create what you will.

— GEORGE BERNARD SHAW

Background

A creative collage, also called an inspiration board or inspiration gallery, is a great tool for sparking creativity. The purpose of the collage is to provide visual cues that will inspire and stimulate you toward your next creative endeavor. When you gaze upon it, the carefully selected items should stir in you the desire to respond in some way. Items on the collage can range from the artfully beautiful to the stylishly whimsical to the boldly innovative. Whatever it is that makes you see the world in a different way, opening you up to new possibilities, is the perfect choice.

Getting Started

Begin by gathering items for your collage in a folder. This step may take some time as it is better to find truly unique and inspiring objects, rather than settling for less exceptional images just to fill the space. Once you are satisfied with your assortment, determine what backing you would like to use to create the collage. If permanently affixing the items, experiment with the layout over a period of time until you are comfortable with the arrangement. If using a bulletin board or magnetized board, you can begin affixing the items immediately, endlessly tweaking the arrangement.

Noteworthy

- There are a number of different surfaces that can be used when creating a collage, including online templates, construction paper, or foam board. Bulletin boards are perfect for creating a collage since items can easily be added or taken away, and are available in a wide array of beautiful colors and frames. When hung above a desk, the collage doubles as a work of art, providing interest in the designated room.

- Don't worry about trying to organize your creative collage around any particular theme or pattern. Oftentimes we choose things that inspire us without specifically knowing why. Over time, ask yourself what it was in each object that demanded your attention.

- You may want to add embellishments to your collage in the form of ribbons, beads, feathers, string, or fabric. A 3-D object will provide the collage additional depth and interest.

Directions: In the coming week, begin collecting items to add to your creative collage. If you are at a loss for where to look, try the following resources:

- ☐ Post cards from an art museum gift shop
- ☐ Architecture, design, and gardening magazines
- ☐ Unique high-end greeting cards like Papyrus
- ☐ Color photocopies of pictures from books
- ☐ Poetry books/websites
- ☐ Websites devoted to creativity, art, design, and inspiration
- ☐ Samples from fabric stores
- ☐ Pictures of unique or creative businesses
- ☐ Online quote websites
- ☐ Bookmarks, gift wrap, and wallpaper samples
- ☐ Photographs or sepia images
- ☐ Outdated calendars
- ☐ Marbleized paper
- ☐ Dried flowers and leaves
- ☐ Antique maps
- ☐ Illuminated manuscripts
- ☐ Portraits of an artist or inventor you admire
- ☐ Album covers
- ☐ Sheet music
- ☐ Magazine articles or newspaper clippings of inspirational individuals

ADDITIONAL NOTES:

VOLUNTEERISM | Helping Yourself By Helping Others

Every good act is charity. A man's true wealth hereafter is the good that he does in this world to his fellows.
— MOLIERE

Background

The history of volunteerism in the United States dates back as early as the 1600s when citizens of colonial New England banded together to form volunteer fire brigades when combating fires. Throughout the Great Awakening of the 19th Century, individuals became increasingly aware of the plight of the disadvantaged and in 1851 the first YMCA was formed. Later, during the American Civil War, Clara Barton and a team of volunteers would work tirelessly to provide aid for servicemen with Barton eventually forming the American Red Cross in 1881. Today volunteerism is woven through the fabric of American culture with more than 68 million volunteers recorded working for various organizations in 2013.

Getting Started

Although unpaid service provides immeasurable good to countless worthy groups within a community, it could be argued that the greatest benefactor of volunteerism is the volunteer herself. The first step to becoming a volunteer is identifying your interests and goals. What causes are you passionate about? How much responsibility are you willing to take on? Do you bring any particular skills to the situation? How much time do you have available to donate? Once you've considered these questions you can begin to narrow prospective opportunities.

Noteworthy

- Measuring a large group of adults in America, researchers at the London School of Economics found the likelihood of being "very happy" rose 7 percent among those who volunteer monthly and 12 percent for individuals who volunteer every couple weeks. This increases to 16 percent for those volunteering weekly with religious organizations having the greatest impact.

- Volunteering not only increases self-confidence and combats depression, but helps you stay physically fit, an important consideration for older adults. Studies found those who volunteer have a lower mortality rate than those who don't, even when other factors are taken into account.

- A side benefit of volunteerism is the ability to advance your career through the acquisition of valuable skills, allowing you to test out a new career without making a long-term commitment. If you are interested in nursing, you might spend a few hours each week in a hospital or assist at an animal shelter if considering a career in animal science.

Directions: Complete the following page to get started volunteering in your community.

1 Where to Look

- **www.getinvolved.gov** and **www.volunteer.gov** will help you locate opportunities
- Community theaters, museums, and monuments
- Libraries or senior centers
- Historical restorations and national parks
- Youth organizations, sports teams, and after-school programs
- Food banks, shelters or Salvation Army
- Places of worship
- Service organizations such as Rotary or Lions Club

2 List Causes You Are Interested in Here:

_____

_____

_____

_____

_____

_____

_____

3 Tips to Keep in Mind

- Spend some time making sure you are a good fit for whatever cause you choose. What have you wanted your whole life to try? Why not attempt it now? Ask questions about your time commitment, whether training is involved, and whom you will be working with so that you know what is expected.
- Think outside the box by looking beyond the typical opportunities that come to mind. Many community groups such as disaster relief programs, prisons, historical preservation societies, blood drives, and political campaigns are looking for volunteers.
- Find the volunteer activity that fits into your schedule since organizations need different levels of commitment. Some will require a regular, intensive commitment while others can be occasional or seasonal.
- Don't be afraid to make a change if your experience isn't what you expected. Talk with the organization about changing your duties or look for another match altogether.
- If you prefer to work from home and have computer skills, consider virtual volunteering by assisting an organization online.

Volunteer Contract

I pledge to donate _____ hours monthly to the following cause(s):

_____

_____

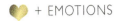

BOLT OF JOY

Pleasure is spread throughout the earth in stray gifts to be claimed by whoever shall find.

— WILLIAM WORDSWORTH

Background

Every morning, we each have the ability to create our own happiness without relying on other people or outside circumstances. Authentic happiness has been defined as contentment with the past, joy in the present, and hope for the future. Throughout this project you will be concentrating on intensifying your joy in the present by accessing the list of pleasures and joys brainstormed in the first week and inserting them into daily practice.

Getting Started

In this week's project you will attempt to move the pleasures and joys that occur in our lives from spontaneous occurrences to intentional daily events. Each morning (or previous evening before retiring to bed), ask yourself what one specific thing you will do that day, no matter how small, to increase your joy. Will you visit your favorite greenhouse, call an old friend, savor a glass of wine, make biscotti, paint a picture, write a card, attend a dance class, scour an antique store, or enjoy a nap?

Noteworthy

- According to the gentleman credited as the founding father of positive psychology, Dr. Martin Seligman, there are three concepts that will help you get the most out of your daily bolts of joy. The first concept is *habituation*, the idea that as humans we adapt surprisingly quickly to most any stimulus. If you treat yourself to a latte every day, it won't produce the same bump in happiness as indulging only occasionally. Vary your joys to keep them fresh and novel.

- The second concept is *savoring*, which implies a heightened sense of delight and thankfulness throughout the experience. You can achieve this more readily by having all of your senses engaged. If you are enjoying a bath, be aware of the sensation of bubbles, the smell of added oil, the sight of a candle nearby, and the sound of the water or soft music.

- The final concept is **mindfulness** or being deliberately attentive throughout the entire experience. This occurs more readily when in a slow state of mind rather than when one's thoughts are racing to the future. If you are getting a pedicure, for instance, do not let the entire 30-minutes slip by while on your phone or otherwise distracted.

Directions: Throughout the week build a bolt of joy into your daily routine by asking yourself what one thing you can do that day to increase your happiness (refer to your *What Makes Me Happy?* list for ideas). In the notes section record a description of the activity, what you did to savor it more fully, or your gratitude for the experience.

BOLT OF JOY:

NOTES: DATE:

BOLT OF JOY:

NOTES: DATE:

BOLT OF JOY:

NOTES: DATE:

BOLT OF JOY:

NOTES: DATE:

BOLT OF JOY:

NOTES: DATE:

BOLT OF JOY:

NOTES: DATE:

BOLT OF JOY:

NOTES: DATE:

ADDITIONAL NOTES:

+ EXPRESSION

(CREATIVITY)

Learn why creativity, inherently present in each of us, is an important component of quality living

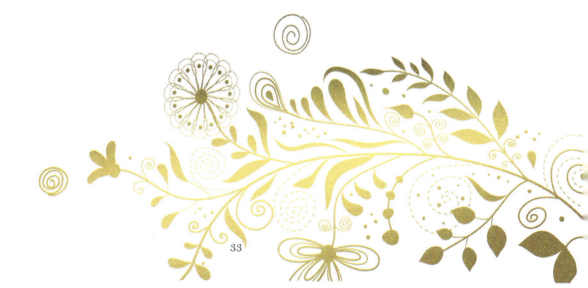

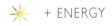

DRINKING FOR ENERGY

Water sustains all.

— THALES OF MILETUS, 600 B.C.

Background

When it comes to fighting fatigue and optimizing energy, consuming adequate water throughout the day is critical. The human body is made up of approximately 60 percent water with the brain made up of a whopping 85 percent. Water affects our energy, flushing toxins from our body, maintaining regularity, and keeping our metabolic system in good working order. Common side effects of dehydration include increased hunger, headaches, lightheadedness, muscle cramps, lowered blood pressure, bloating, and difficulty concentrating.

Getting Started

Although we're all familiar with the recommended eight, eight-ounce glasses rule for daily consumption, a more customized way to determine daily intake is to drink half your body weight in ounces. It's a good idea to consume one to two of those glasses upon waking and one prior to each meal. Find a system to help you remember how much you've drank throughout the day. This can be done by filling a large container with the entire amount at the beginning of the day, using tally marks on your phone, having a glass after each trip to the restroom, drinking during transitional times (upon waking, at breakfast, when sitting down to work, etc.), or simply having a glass every hour on the hour until you've met your quota.

Noteworthy

* It is believed nearly 80 percent of headaches are caused by dehydration, and it is thought to be a trigger for migraines. A common symptom of dehydration headaches is an increase in pain when moving the head — especially when walking. It is believed the blood vessels in the head may actually narrow in an attempt to regulate body fluids.

* A study by the University of North Carolina at Chapel Hills revealed that those who drink water regularly consume about 200 fewer calories a day than those who only drink tea, coffee, or soda. That works out to a loss of nearly 21 pounds a year.

* When considering daily water intake don't forget the following hydration robbers: alcohol, sodium, cabin pressure while flying, certain medications, extremely hot/dry/cold climates, illness, and exercise.

Directions: Consider the following ideas to make your water drinking routine a more enjoyable experience or experiment with your own concoctions.

Ice Cube Ideas:

- Freeze clementine slices
- Thread a trio of berries onto a toothpick and freeze
- Add bits of orange, lemon, and lime peel
- Freeze chunks of pineapple
- Fill ice cube tray with unsweetened juice

Flavorful Combinations to Add to Your Water:

- Lemon + lime + orange slices
- Apple slices + cinnamon sticks
- Strawberry + lime + mint
- Lavender + lime wedge
- Cucumber + ginger slices + mint
- Lime + cucumber + basil
- Watermelon chunks + rosemary
- Grapefruit + basil

Additional Ideas:

- Get a home seltzer maker (i.e. Soda Stream) to add fizz to your H2O.
- Add a splash of unsweetened cranberry or apple juice to your water.
- Instead of your first cup of coffee in the morning try hot water with a squeeze of lemon juice.
- Purchase a pretty drinking glass and straws, which help you to take in more liquid at a time.
- Keep a bottle in your car for those times you're waiting in line at a bank or pharmacy.

NOTES:

ANNUAL LEARNING GOAL

Develop a passion for learning. If you do, you will never cease to grow.

— ANTHONY J. D'ANGELO

Background

It is well documented that continuous life-long learning, particularly in subject areas that are of deep personal interest and fairly challenging, can go a long ways toward the delay of cognitive problems as we age. A 2004 study by researchers at Rush Medical Center in Chicago found that higher levels of education help build a *cognitive reserve* within the brain that helps protect against dementia. Perhaps more important than years of formal education per se is support for ongoing participation through cognitively stimulating activities.

Getting Started

Committing to an annual learning goal goes a long way to ensuring you stay intellectually stimulated throughout your life. Goals in a variety of areas are essential for keeping us headed in the right direction and are a proven strategy for becoming lastingly happier. Brainstorm ideas for a stimulating learning goal you can focus on in the coming year. This might include taking up a new instrument (or returning to an abandoned one), learning a second language, enrolling in art history classes at your community college, or creating a blog on a particular interest. Keep in mind the goal should be intrinsically meaningful and authentic to your personal pursuits.

Noteworthy

◎ Though it may seem counterintuitive, it is the striving for goals that appears to make people happier rather than the actual attainment of a goal. The primary purpose of a future goal is present-day happiness.

◎ Choose a SMART goal using the following guidelines:

S – Specific goals are clearly defined verbally and in writing
M – Measureable goals achieve better effort and results
A – Attainable goals are challenging, but doable
R – Relevant goals are deeply personal and self-concordant
T – Time-based goals include a time-line and can be tracked

Directions: Choose a learning goal that you would take great personal interest and pleasure in attaining in the coming year.

GOAL

Steps or Action Plan for accomplishing goal including timeline:

1.

2.

3.

4.

5.

6.

Potential obstacles for achieving goal:

What materials, outside expertise, or support do I require to be succesful?

_____

_____

_____

_____

_____

_____

_____

_____

_____

_____

_____

_____

_____

_____

_____

_____

My goal is: NOTES:

_____ Specific and clearly defined

_____ Measureable

_____ Challenging

_____ Attainable

_____ Meaningful / relevant

_____ Time-based

ADDITIONAL NOTES:

STOMP THE ANTS

It takes but one positive thought when given a chance to survive and thrive to overpower an entire army of negative thoughts.

— ROBERT H. SCHULLER

Background

Automatic Negative Thoughts (ANTS) are unproductive phrases or sentences that seep into our consciousness without warning. Often we are not even aware of their presence, but they have a tremendous impact on our quality of life. It was Aaron Beck and Albert Ellis in the 1970s who argued what we consciously think about affects how we feel. From their thesis *Behavior Cognitive Therapy* emerged as a way to combat negative thinking about failure, defeat, loss, and helplessness. It was discovered that by replacing negative thoughts with more optimistic ones, individuals were better equipped to achieve resiliency and happiness.

Getting Started

Dr. Daniel Amen, author of *Change Your Brain, Change Your Body*, identified different types of ANTs that infiltrate our thinking and developed corresponding ANT-eater solutions to use when you catch yourself in one of these negative thinking patterns. As soon as you find yourself thinking in an unproductive way, you need to stomp the ANT. This can be done in a number of ways. Even saying the word STOP forcibly can be enough to break the mental cycle. For the purpose of this exercise you will be asked to wear a slip-on bracelet on your wrist in the coming week. Once you identify a negative thought and replace it with a more positive one using the techniques on the following page, move the bangle to the opposite wrist. After twenty-one days of not having to move the bangle the pattern should be reversed.

Noteworthy

- The average person has approximately 60,000 thoughts per day. Nearly 95 percent of those thoughts are repetitive in nature (you thought about them the day before and the day before that). Even more sobering is the fact that up to 80 percent are negative.

- CBT is still widely used today and often recommended for those suffering from insomnia to help reset negative thinking that accompanies sleeping issues.

- You may wish to carry a notebook with you, writing down examples of negative thinking as they occur ("I look fat in this outfit," "I hate being stuck in traffic," "I wish it would quit raining") and tallying the results at the end of each day. Look for patterns such as when negative thoughts are most likely to occur.

Directions: Purchase an inexpensive stretch bracelet to represent a particularly pesky, negative thought pattern. Use the suggested ANT-eater to replace the thought and bangle.

TYPES OF NEGATIVE THINKING

1. **All or Nothing:** In this type of black and white thinking, things are seen as either all good or all bad. This distorted thinking leads you to believe because you slipped once on your diet, you might as well give up.
   ANT-eater: Acknowledge that one slip up doesn't mean your diet is ruined. Start again the next day.

2. **Using "always," "never," "every time," "everyone":** Broad generalizations using these words, (*"Everyone gets invited out on Friday night but me"*) can cause depression and lead to anxiety.
   ANT-eater: Ban over-generalized words, which are never accurate. Not everyone is going out on Friday so be proactive and plan an outing with a friend.

3. **Fortune Telling:** This is predicting the worse even when you don't know what is going to happen (*"I bet this new mole is skin cancer"*). This form of ANT is particularly common and can manifest rapidly unless you take control.
   ANT-eater: No one can predict the future and most of the things we worry about never materialize. What can be a problem is chronic stress from worry, which has been linked to a number of diseases.

4. **Labeling:** Labeling (*"I'm so clueless with technology"*) is always unproductive. Once a person begins to believe their negative labels, they are more likely to have a defeatist attitude, giving up easily in tough situations.
   ANT-eater: Avoid putting labels on yourself and others. Flip any negative labels you already have. ("It might take me awhile to figure out new technology, but I always get it eventually.")

5. **Mind Reading:** When you believe you know what someone else is thinking you are mind reading. (*"I know my co-worker thinks I'm not doing a good job."*) We often ruminate about what someone else might be thinking when in truth we have no idea what he or she thinks.
   ANT-eater: Don't assume you know what others think.

6. **Blaming Others:** This toxic ANT makes you a victim and keeps you from taking responsibility for your own successes and failures. It is always easier to blame others for difficult circumstances, but will ultimately make you unhappy.
   ANT-eater: Regardless of what someone else has done to you in the past, resolve to be in charge of your own destiny.

7. **Guilt:** Using words such as "should," "must," "ought," and "have to" allow feelings of guilt to build up and begin affecting your behavior adversely.
   ANT-eater: Avoid labeling yourself in the future, and correct any existing labels you secretly harbor. ("I am not lazy and worthless.")

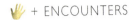

FOR THE LOVE OF FRIENDS

But if the while I think on thee, dear friend, All losses are restored and sorrows end.
— WILLIAM SHAKESPEARE

Background

Although Valentine's Day began as a celebration of the early Christian Saint Valentine who performed weddings for young soldiers against the wishes of Claudius II, the day was first associated with romantic love during the Middle Ages, where the tradition of courtly love flourished. In 17th-century England it evolved into an occasion where lovers expressed their affection to one another by offering cards, sweets, and flowers. Handmade Valentine cards made of lace and ribbons, featuring cupids and hearts, eventually spread to the American colonies.

Getting Started

With a beautiful color palette (pinks, reds, gold, and silver), delectable candy confections, and every imaginable form of greeting card, Valentine's Day is far too enticing a holiday to reserve for just one person. Why not make it a day to celebrate your friendships as well as your romantic partner? Some time within the first two weeks of February, plan a special recognition of your closest friends using one of the ideas shared on the following page or choosing one of your own. Your efforts will be particularly appreciated by those friends without a love interest, but equally in need of being cherished during the dark, dreary days of February.

Noteworthy

- Red roses became known as the favored flower for love because it was the favorite flower of Venus, Goddess of Love. Juggling the letters of the word ROSE results in EROS, God of Love.

- In Finland Valentine's Day is called Ystävänpäivä, which translates to "Friend's Day" and is more about remembering your friends than loved ones.

- The expression "wear your heart on your sleeve" came from the Middle Ages when a young man or women would choose a paper heart from a bowl with a name on it and pin it to their sleeves for a week to express their affection.

- In Victorian times it was considered bad luck to sign a Valentine's Day card.

Directions: Choose one of the following ideas for celebrating your friendships or come up with one of your own.

Create a Card

Let your creativity soar with an over-the-top card that resembles a miniature work of art when complete. Think Victorian with bits of lace, gold leaf, 3-D elements, fancy calligraphy, and sealing wax. In the greeting include your favorite attribute of that friend and the reason they are so special to you.

For inspiration check out the archives of the Graceful Envelope Contest held annually by the Washington (DC) Calligraphy Guild at calligraphersguild.org.

Give a Gift

- Fill a jar with brightly colored candy, add a touch of glitter to the top of the lid, and tie on a tag with raffia

- Bake cranberry biscotti drizzled with white chocolate and fill a decorative bag tied with ribbon.

- Make a homemade body scrub and place in a pretty glass container with small wooden scoop tied to the lid.

- Place a picture of the two of you in a small heart frame.

Host at Home

Create a special occasion for your friends by hosting an afternoon or evening Valentine Dessert Buffet. Purchase or make 3–4 tempting desserts and display them on a sideboard or serving table decorated with a gold runner, variety of candles, and beautiful flowers.

ADDITIONAL NOTES:

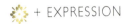

HABITS OF HIGHLY CREATIVE PEOPLE

There is a fountain of youth: it is your mind, your talents, the creativity you bring to your life and the lives of people you love. When you learn to tap this source, you will truly have defeated age.

— SOPHIA LOREN

Background

Creativity is a mysterious and often elusive commodity where, at times, we find inspiration almost out of nowhere and other times we cannot call it forth no matter what we do. It has proven to be more complex than we once believed when individuals were either pegged as left brained (analytical and rational) or right brained (creative and emotional). In fact, creativity is now thought to involve a number of cognitive processes, neural pathways, and emotions. In trying to form a profile of creative people, we find they are difficult to summarize because they tend to avoid habit and routine. Research suggests creativity involves a number of factors, which together influence the individual.

Getting Started

While there's no "typical" creative type, there are some distinguishing characteristics behaviors attributed to highly creative people. If you consider yourself creative or you work frequently in the arts, you may recognize some of these habits in yourself. If you do not identify with the concept of creativity, you might benefit from incorporating some of these habits into your daily routine. Most of them require nothing more than an awareness of how to approach life differently.

Noteworthy

- Do not give up on creative endeavors because you do not produce the perfect product or even a product you are happy with. Resiliency goes hand and hand with creative endeavors. Successful creative types do not take failure personally, but learn to fail repeatedly until they find what works for them.

- Creative individuals are keen observers of other humans, watching them intently in a variety of situations and locations. The next time you are in a coffee shop or airport, put down your reading material or electronic device and watch the humanity humming along around you.

- All creative endeavors involve risk. "There is a deep and meaningful connection between risk taking and creativity and it's one that's often overlooked," Steven Kotler wrote in *Forbes*. "Creativity is the act of making something for nothing. It requires making public those bets first placed by imagination. This is not a job for the timid."

Directions: Consider the following habits of creative people as compiled by New York University psychologist Scott Barry Kaufman, who spent years researching creativity. Keep this sheet in front of you this week to remind you of ways to encourage your creative nature.

1. **They observe everything:** The creative person sees possibilities everywhere and is continually absorbing information from the world around them to be used at another time. A journal kept on hand is perfect for taking notes on all that stirs the imagination.

2. **They work the hours that work for them:** Individuals with high creative potential figure out what time they work best and structure their day accordingly. Determine what time of day you are most productive and reserve a portion of it forcreative endeavors.

3. **They take time for solitude:** If every minute of your day is scheduled, it's difficult to get in touch with your inner creative voice. You need moments of solitude to let your mind wander, to daydream. Allow yourself time to sit outside with no agenda other than to drift.

4. **They turn life's obstacles around:** Creative people use periods of suffering as catalysts for substantial creative growth. Researchers have found trauma can help people to grow in the areas of interpersonal relationships, spirituality, appreciation of life, and personal strength as well as creativity. Can you think of a silver lining that came from a difficult situation?

5. **They seek out new experiences:** Creative people love to expose themselves to new experiences, sensations, and states of mind. "Openness to experience is consistently the strongest indicator of creative achievement," says Kaufman. Set an intention to experience one new activity this month.

6. **They ask the big questions:** Creative people are unrelentingly curious. They choose to live the examined life and, as they age, they continue to maintain a curiosity about life. They look around them and want to know why and how. What one thing comes to mind that you'd like to know more about?

7. **They follow their true passions:** Creative people tend to be intrinsically motivated and are energized by challenging activities. "Eminent creators choose and become passionately involved in challenging, risky problems that provide a powerful sense of power from the ability to use their talents," write M.A. Collins and T. M. Amabile.

8. **They lose track of time:** Creative types tend to lose themselves in their projects, transcending time with activities that they are good at, but which also challenge them. What activities or projects draw you in and cause you to lose track of time?

9. **They surround themselves with beauty:** Creative individuals are naturally drawn to beauty and surround themselves accordingly. Be on the look out for items of beauty from nature or art that will inspire you each time you gaze upon them.

10. **They connect the dots:** If there's one thing that distinguishes highly creative people from others, it's the ability to see possibilities where others don't – to have a vision. Make an effort to look at projects and situations you encounter from different perspectives.

ADDITIONAL NOTES:

IT TAKES A VILLAGE

If we are to teach real peace in this world, and if we are to carry on a real war against war, we shall have to begin with the children.

— MOHANDAS GANDHI

Background

How often do you get the chance to change the course of someone's life for the better? All across the globe reside children living in substandard conditions for reasons ranging from malnutrition to lack of education to the need for appropriate role models. Decide what you can do for a child in need whether it be a financial donation or donation of time. In most communities there are homeless shelters, after-school programs, and at-risk teenager programs. If you are new to the area, United Way has a large list of charities that specialize in helping disadvantaged children. You may wish to become a Big Brother/Big Sister, which allows you to interact with a child in need of additional attention with as little as four hours of your time monthly. Or you may choose the ultimate gift to give a child in need — becoming a foster parent.

Getting Started

The first step in determining how you are able to contribute to the well being of a disadvantaged child is considering what areas speak to you most. Are you more passionate about issues of hunger, housing, literacy, or abuse? Once you've determined an interest, spend sufficient time researching related organizations in your community and on a national or global stage. Be sure you understand the commitment involved in terms of both time and money. In the case of sponsoring a child, you may be asked to fulfill that obligation until the child reaches a certain age, often eighteen years.

Noteworthy

- According to UNICEF, 22,000 children die each day due to poverty and 2.2 million children die each year because they are not immunized. Of the 1.9 billion children from the developing world, 1 in 3 are without adequate shelter and 1 in 5 without access to safe water.

- Every day, within the United States 1,900 children become victims of abuse or neglect, and four of them will die.

- Less than 1 percent of what the world spends every year on weapons is needed to put every child in the world in school.

Directions: Use the following ideas to determine how you might help a child in your community or in a developing country.

Help feed children

- Sponsor a child for a low monthly cost to ensure minimum dietary requirements and basic education from respected organizations such as *World Vision*, *Save the Children*, or *Compassion International*.
- Launch a virtual food drive by setting up a page through *Feeding America*, setting a target goal, and asking friends and family to donate using the online tools provided.
- Consider volunteering on a larger scale with international organizations such as *Feed My Starving Children* or *Feed the Children*.
- Volunteer at local churches, women's shelters, or community centers that provide sack lunches or weekly meals to disadvantaged families.

Help tutor children

- Volunteer at a Title I school within your community with children who would benefit from additional face time with an adult.
- *United Way Volunteer Readers* matches volunteers to read with students, asking for a commitment of an hour a week.
- Online tutoring is another option that allows greater flexibility.

Help disabled children

- *The Arc* is one of the world's largest disability organizations with more than 140,000 members in 780 chapters. Volunteer opportunities exist at most local chapters; simply contact for more information.
- *Special Olympics* is always in need of volunteers to help in a variety of ways during competitions.
- Help raise money or volunteer with *Children's Relief Fund* to fund therapy, equipment, summer programs, and other group activities for disabled children.

Help abused children

- One of the best things you can do to help abused children is report abuse by contacting local law enforcement as soon as possible.
- *Childhelp* is a well known organization that works to promote child advocacy, abuse prevention and treatment, as well as community outreach.
- CASA (*Court Appointed Special Advocates*) is a network of 951 communitybased programs that recruit, train, and support volunteers to advocate for the best interests of abused and neglected children in courtrooms and communities.

MY GOAL TO HELP CHILDREN IN MY COMMUNITY OR AROUND THE WORLD:

....

....

....

THREE GOOD THINGS

"What day is it?" "It's today," squeaked Piglet. "My favorite day," said Pooh.

— A.A. MILNE

Background

The benefits of optimism – the idea that while there are sure to be ups and downs in life, overall things will work out in the end – are as varied as they are numerous. Optimists enjoy greater health, perform better athletically and academically, are more likely to achieve financial success because they don't give up, maintain better mental health, experience less stress, and demonstrate increased life longevity. At its core, optimism leads people to make healthy, constructive choices that bring about favorable results. If you tend to be excited about the future, believing you will enjoy your grandchildren into old age, you are more likely to follow through with behaviors – like eating well and exercising – that help make that a reality. If, on the other hand, you harbor gloomier predictions of the future, you may tell yourself it doesn't matter when indulging in unhealthy behaviors.

Getting Started

For this project you will be asked each evening to record three good things that happened throughout that day. Maybe you completed a big project or the cold you thought you were getting didn't materialize or you found the perfect parking spot in front of the grocery store. It is a mental recording of the positive experiences you encountered no matter how seemingly insignificant. This is particularly powerful on your lowest days because it makes you more aware, even then, that something good is bound to have happened during the day. At its core, it is training the brain to look at the glass as half full. If optimism does not come naturally to you, take comfort knowing it is a skill that can be improved and strengthened with time.

Noteworthy

- This exercise is similar, but different, from recording those things you are grateful for in a gratitude list. Rather than focusing on specific blessings in your life, you are objectively noting the random positive happenings that are scattered throughout each of our days.

- Research carried out by scientists who studied 100,000 women deduced that women who were generally pessimistic had higher blood pressure and cholesterol while optimistic women had a 9 percent lower risk of developing heart disease and a 14 percent lower risk of dying from any cause after more than eight years of follow-up.

- Optimists are more proactive with stress management, favoring approaches that reduce or eliminate stressors and their emotional consequences. Optimists work harder at stress management, so they're less stressed. They see negative events as minor set backs to be overcome.

Directions: Start the habit of jotting down at least three positive things that happened to you throughout the day. You might choose to do this in the evening as you are preparing for sleep.

SUNDAY
1.
2.
3.

MONDAY
1.
2.
3.

TUESDAY
1.
2.
3.

WEDNESDAY
1.
2.
3.

THURSDAY
1.
2.
3.

FRIDAY
1.
2.
3.

SATURDAY
1.
2.
3.

EATING FOR ENERGY

Nothing would be more tiresome than eating and drinking if God had not made them a pleasure as well as a necessity.

— VOLTAIRE

Background

While most of us are aware of the fact that what we eat impacts how we feel, many people don't realize how substantially food can affect our energy level, sometimes in as little as a few hours. That is because most of what we read regarding food focuses on losing weight rather than maximizing energy. Begin your journey toward healthier eating by first becoming familiar with the top power foods. Included within this illustrious group are such foods as eggs, yogurt, salmon, almonds, beans, spinach and kale, apples, berries, broccoli, dark chocolate, walnuts, garlic, and avocados. From there, begin familiarizing yourself with the food guidelines on the following page to ensure your food choices keep you revved throughout the day.

Getting Started

Tracking your energy levels throughout the day is the best way to figure out how different types of food affect you. Keep a simple log of the foods you eat and corresponding energy over the next 3–4 hours. Before long, patterns will start to emerge such as: Ate a high protein breakfast this morning; didn't feel hungry or tired all morning. Consider the suggestions on the following page to determine effects on your daily energy.

Noteworthy

* For maximum energy, eat foots low on the glycemic index. This is a useful guide for determining how quickly the food you eat is turned into glucose. High GI foods such as white bread, white rice, cereals, and baked goods are easily converted to glucose in your body. Low GI food such as most vegetables, meat, milk, nuts, and eggs are converted more slowly.

* Consider your eating schedule for the day like a pyramid with breakfast large and filling and your evening snack the tiny top. In addition to increasing your early morning calorie intake and decreasing your evening intake, you need to incorporate protein throughout the day. Nearly all cases of mid-morning blahs or afternoon fatigue can be attributed to low blood sugar.

* Although there is wide discussion as to how often you should eat, try not to go more than four hours without food. This allows for three small meals and I – 2 snacks. This will keep your blood sugar steady and energy stable throughout the day. Large meals demand more of your energy to digest and can leave you feeling lethargic.

Directions: Strive to become familiar with the following suggestions taken from the book *S.A.S.S! Yourself Slim* for eating to maximize energy.

Eat more iron from plants: Iron is needed to deliver oxygen to cells. Too little of it can cause fatigue, impair physical and mental endurance, and decrease immunity. The best source of iron is through a plant-based diet rich in such food sources as beans, lentils, spinach, and sesame seeds. Eating them with vitamin-C rich foods can boost iron absorption.

Eat the right food combinations: The right combination for maximum energy is fruit or vegetable + whole grain + lean protein + plant based fat + herb/spice. Because your body likes to be in balance, giving it less of something it needs throws things off, as does giving it more than it needs.

Skip the caffeine: Despite health benefits of tea and coffee, if you're feeling run down, you may choose to cut this from your diet. Because caffeine is a stimulant it will give you an initial boost of energy, but may leave you more tired afterwards.

Eat an energizing breakfast: Instead of just having yogurt, add some high antioxidant fruit, good fat such as nuts or seeds and raw or toasted oats. You may wish to try organic nonfat yogurt to maximize protein and quality.

Eat more real food: Eating food that is closer to nature will pay off big dividends in terms of energy. Eat whole grains rather than processed chips or crackers from a box, whole fruit rather than juice or bars, lean cuts of meat rather than hot dogs or chicken nuggets.

Eat more superfruits: Eat a wide variety of superfruits including apples, stone fruits, berries, and tomatoes rather than the same daily banana. Research shows that people who eat a wider variety of fruit have less oxidative stress, which is a precursor to aging and disease.

Avoid the energy trap: Avoid those foods that can zap energy including processed and artificial foods, refined grains and sugar. Also, avoid skipping meals, and drinking too much caffeine and alcohol.

Eat good fats: Don't eliminate fat if you want more energy. Some antioxidants have to grab onto fat in order to be absorbed from the gastrointestinal tract to the blood, where it goes to work. Antioxidants are important for energy because they send free radicals, which can damage cells by altering their structure, running and keep your cells healthy.

Eat in season: Nutritionists will tell you to eat locally and in season. When you go to your farmers markets, the food is often harvested less than 48 hours before you buy it. And because it didn't travel far, it was allowed to reach its peak, which means more nutrients.

Choose frozen food: When you can't get fresh food locally, frozen foods are a potent source of energizing nutrients. Freezing actually locks in nutrients, so a frozen fruit or vegetable with no added ingredients can be just as nutritious as fresh.

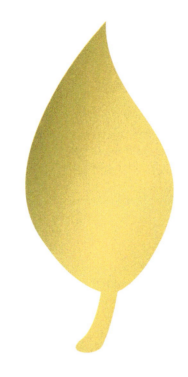

+ EARTH

(GREATER GOOD)

*Uncover ways to positively impact your community,
the nation, and our planet*

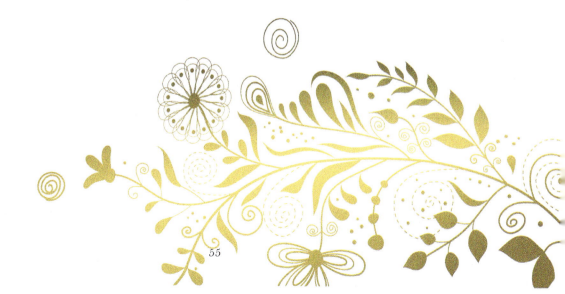

FLOW

It is your passion that empowers you to be able to do that thing you were created to do.

— T. D. JAKES

Background

In the 1970s Hungarian-born researcher Mihaly Csikszentmihalyi (pronounced cheeks-sent-me-high) of Claremont University introduced the concept of flow, the mental state in which a person is fully immersed in an activity to the exclusion of all outside distractions. Flow consists of "optimal experiences" that produce powerful enjoyment, creativity, and total involvement. Consider a runner trying to beat his own record, a cellist mastering an intricate passage, or a bridge player devising the perfect strategy. During flow people become so swept up in what they are doing it is difficult to separate their being from the actions and time appears to "stand still."

Getting Started

Contrary to what we typically believe, the most rewarding moments of our lives are not passive or relaxing times, but occur when a person's body or mind is stretched to its limits in a voluntary effort to accomplish something difficult and worthwhile. You may be one of the lucky individuals who finds herself frequently in flow, whether at work or home. But if you would like to elevate more of your activities into flow experiences, study the sample on the following page.

Noteworthy

- The flow experience usually occurs when we confront tasks we have a chance of completing with clear goals and immediate feedback. In creative activities without clear goals, the person must develop a strong personal sense of the intended outcome.

- Working individuals achieve the flow experience (deep concentration, high and balanced challenges, a sense of control and satisfaction) about four times as often at their job than at home in a passive activity such as watching TV.

- Individuals who experience frequent flow experiences in their life score high in the area of life satisfaction even when other key areas such as social connections are deficient or absent.

- One of most frequently mentioned characteristics of flow is the absence of negative or unproductive thinking during the activity. The mind is so focused on the job at hand it allows no room for random unpleasant thoughts.

Directions: Answer the following questions to create additional flow experiences in your everyday life.

1. What is it you do where time seems to "stand still?" List all interests, hobbies, and passions that intrinsically draw you in?

_____

_____

_____

_____

_____

_____

_____

2. Brainstorm how you can encourage flow experiences from these enjoyments (i.e. if you like to garden you could peruse gardening magazines and create a collage, draw a to-scale plan of your ideal garden, join a gardening club, try planting a particular flower you've never attempted before, keep a gardening journal, or make notecards from pressed flowers grown in your garden).

_____

_____

_____

_____

_____

3. Choose one specific area to write a challenging yet attainable goal that provides some type of immediate feedback (i.e. I will be able to complete my entire weight lifting class using 10-15 pound weights within the next six weeks).

_____

_____

_____

_____

_____

LAUGHTER TREASURE TROVE

There is nothing in the world so irresistibly contagious as laughter and good humor.
— MAHATMA GANDHI

Background

In 1979 famous journalist and political peace advocate, Norman Cousins, wrote the book *Anatomy of an Illness as Perceived by the Patient*, detailing his struggle with Marie- Strumpell disease. Told he had little chance of surviving, Cousins developed a recovery program incorporating massive amounts of vitamin C and a positive attitude. This included training himself to laugh to Marx Brothers films, which he claimed gave him two hours of pain-free sleep. Today, Laughter Clubs and Laughter Yoga are gaining popularity. They involve groups of individuals practicing fake laughter together, which eventually becomes genuine. Deep spontaneous laughter provides oxygen to the lungs and brain in the same manner as deep diaphragmatic breathing.

Getting Started

This project is ongoing in nature and at its root simply requires an awareness of what makes you laugh. Anytime you come across a piece of memorabilia that produces feelings of mirth, put it in a decorative box that you designate as your personal Laughter Treasure Trove. Items may include funny pictures or photos of a time you were particularly goofy, an amusing article or comic strip, a piece of clothing, or your child's photo which conjures silly antics, or the program from a comedic play or musical.

Noteworthy

- Physical benefits of laughter include a decrease in stress hormones and increase in infection-fighting antibodies; release of endorphins for an overall sense of wellbeing and relief of pain; as well as an increase of blood flow and function of blood vessels.

- Emotional benefits include a reduction of stress and increase of energy as well as a lessening of negative emotions such as anxiety, anger, and sadness. When humor enters into a difficult situation, it shifts your perspective so that reality appears less threatening.

- Laughter has a number of social benefits as well, strengthening our relationships with family and friends. Sharing laughter and play with others adds joy, vitality, and resilience to our social bonds.

Directions: Over the coming week become more aware of the extent laughter plays in your daily life. Start assembling a Laughter Treasure Trove with items that bring a smile to your face for days you are feeling blue.

Ticket stub to comedy night with friends

Prop from a fun theme or costume party (i.e. hat, glasses, or mask)

One or two favorite funny DVDs that never fail to make you laugh

Journal of hilarious things your child, spouse, or friends have said

Satirical comedy strip
or
witty magazine article

Invite to Bachelorette Party
or
Bunco night with the girls

Silly photo of child of family member

Score card from game night with family or friends

Photo doing something stupid to remind you not to take yourself too seriously

ADDITIONAL NOTES:

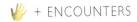

JOIN A SPIRITUAL COMMUNITY

Friendship has always belonged to the core of my spiritual journey.

— HENRI NOUWEN

Background

Spirituality is often defined as a "search for the sacred" and refers to the quest for meaning in life through something that is larger than the individual self. Research has found spiritual people to be happier than nonspiritual people with better mental health, lower mortality, increased ability to deal with chronic disease, happier marriages, and better coping mechanisms during difficult times. These documented benefits are not only the result of lifestyle habits, but also the positive impact of well-established social circles that provide support and reduce stress in a person's life.

Getting Started

Some individuals have never attended church of any type, some have left religion due to previous negative experiences, and some have let the practice go by the wayside due to increasingly busy schedules. Whether or not you choose to be associated with any particular religious institution, you may wish to explore participation in some type of spiritual community. This can be achieved in a number of ways and tailored to fit your particular lifestyle, comfort level, and belief system. Groups founded on spiritual practices provide hope and encouragement to members while fostering greater compassion and assistance for our fellow mankind.

Noteworthy

- An exhaustive review found that people with a strong spiritual life had an 18 percent reduction in mortality, which was comparable to eating a high amount of fruits and vegetables or taking blood pressure medication. Other benefits include a sense of purpose, greater connection to the world, reduced stress through release of control, and expanded support network.

- All major religions including Christianity, Islam, Buddhism, and Judaism emphasize a core belief of forgiveness. Letting go of negative feelings through forgiveness has been linked to numerous health benefits including improved immune function, longer lifespan, lowered blood pressure, and better cardiovascular health.

- People who practice a religion or faith are less likely to smoke, drink, commit a crime, or become involved in a violent activity. They are also more likely to engage in preventative habits such as wearing a seatbelt and taking vitamins.

Directions: Look over the options below for ideas of how you might become more involved in a spiritual community and check those of interest.

_____ Sign up for a meditation or yoga class (check your community calendar for all-day workshops or retreats).

_____ Join a small group or Bible study offered at the church of your choice.

_____ Walk a prayer circle with others.

_____ Sing with a choir (many churches offer both traditional and contemporary services).

_____ Go on a weekend retreat with others (offered to different women or couples groups in many churches).

_____ Gather with friends to listen to the words of inspired speakers such as Martin Luther King.

_____ Light advent or Hanukkah candles during holidays with family members.

_____ Start a prayer group with like-minded individuals to offer one another support and pray for specific concerns.

_____ Participate in church-sponsored charities such as house builds, neighborhood clean ups, weekly meals for the homeless, or Christmas boxes for the needy.

_____ Take regular nature hikes with friends during which you each share what you're grateful for amid the beauty of the outdoors.

_____ Plan a pilgrimage with other women or couples to a shrine or other location of importance to your beliefs.

_____ Join an online spiritual community.

_____ Start a writing group with the theme of your own personal spiritual journeys and share with one another regularly.

_____ Learn about the major world religions in a community college class.

_____ Practice random acts of kindness throughout the week and share your experiences with a small group.

_____ Start a book club that focuses on themes of spirituality.

_____ Initiate a fun ritual by inviting a small group to coffee and scones following church service to discuss that week's message.

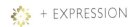

REFRAMING: CREATIVE PROBLEM SOLVING

I never made one of my discoveries from the process of rational thinking.

— ALBERT EINSTEIN

Background

Reframing is the process of altering our perspective of a problem, event, person, project, or situation in order to arrive at a better solution or different end result. When you see an opportunity hidden within a difficult circumstance or view an annoying person in a different light, you are reframing. In its simplest form it involves starting out looking at something one way and ending up seeing it as something else entirely. By trading frames and thus the way you feel, you discover more options and an increased opportunity for action. It allows you to achieve greater clarity when faced with a challenging problem by enhancing your creative thinking to arrive at an innovative solution.

Getting Started

As you go through this week, begin to think of how you can reframe the prickly problems you encounter into more positive situations. If your dated home makes you wish for the hundredth time you could afford to remodel, think about how comfortable people seem to be when they gather there. If the procrastination tendencies of your free-spirited child are driving you crazy, remind yourself of their incredible compassion for others. If you are frustrated with the fact you haven't been going to the gym often enough, try concentrating on how well you've been eating. Switching your focus to the positive things you're doing will free up exhausting negative mental energy. It might just be the boost you need to get back into the gym.

Noteworthy

- Reframing is common in business where the process is used to determine how to remarket a product that hasn't been selling well, how to better utilize employees, or how to rethink an original design.

- Another benefit of reframing is that it increases our empathy and compassion for others. By trying to understand what motivates our friends and family from their point of view rather than only from our own, we strengthen our connections.

- A good way to begin reframing a problem is to start by asking "why." If you are frustrated with a general lack of communication from your boss, ask why. If the answer is you can't tell whether you are doing an appropriate job, ask your boss whether you might meet monthly for a few minutes to touch base on current projects.

Directions: Using the following questions as creative frames of reference, work through a particularly difficult problem or situation to arrive at a different frame of mind.

Name a problem or situation that currently has you frustrated or feeling "stuck."

How does this problem affect you personally?

What do you most want or need to happen in this situation?

Try to put yourself in the shoes of the other people involved. What do you believe their thinking might be with regard to this situation?

Do you need to call upon outside individuals or resources for assistance?

_____

_____

_____

_____

List two possible reframes for this situation.

_____

_____

_____

_____

What steps can you take at this point to begin turning the situation around?

_____

_____

_____

_____

What is one positive outcome or new opportunity that could potentially result from this situation?

_____

_____

_____

_____

ADDITIONAL NOTES:

SHOP FAIRTRADE

You have not lived today until you have done something for someone who can never repay you.
— JOHN BUNYAN

Background

Fairtrade (Fair Trade) began as a grassroots movement of conscious consumers and companies working with farmers around the world to push for trade on more equal terms. To date more than 27,000 products sold in more than 120 countries carry the Fairtrade mark. Within the international mark, the blue sky represents potential and is connected to the green of new growth with the silhouette of a person raising an arm in celebration of the human endeavor. Purchase of products with the mark ensures ongoing support for Fairtrade farmers and workers in the field and the development of the internationally agreed upon Fairtrade standards, minimum prices, and premiums.

Getting Started

The international Fairtrade mark and Fair Trade USA mark are showing up on the shelves of co-ops, grocery stores, and specialty shops across the U.S. Every choice you make while wandering the shopping aisle is your chance to help make a difference for smallscale farmers and workers located around the world. Help increase the Fair Trade impact by spreading the word to friends and family, joining a campaign in your area, and frequenting those businesses that support these organizations.

Noteworthy

- Most fair trade organizations are members of or certified by one of several national or international federations with Fairtrade International being the largest and most widely recognized. In America, the organization is known as Fair Trade USA with a logo showing the black silhouette of a person holding a basket.

- For those products with single ingredients (i.e. coffee or bananas), 100 percent of the product has met the Fairtrade standards. For composite products (i.e. cookies, ice cream, and chocolate bars), all ingredients that can be sourced as Fairtrade must be Fairtrade.

- A number of companies provide products with the Fairtrade mark including: Ben & Jerry's, Wonder Food Co, Starbucks Coffee Co, Divine Chocolate, BloomQuest, Green & Black's Organic Chocolate, Lily's Sweets, Nielsen-Massey Vanillas, Steep & Brew, Verve, and Vittoria Coffee USA.

Directions: Using the following product guide, make an effort this week to locate shops and stores in your community that sell Fair Trade items.

FAIR TRADE PRODUCT GUIDE

Coffee and Tea: Coffee was the original Fair Trade product and there are almost 500 brands available in North America today. In addition to ground and whole bean, you are likely to find the label on k-cups as well. Fair Trade tea is also available, both bagged and loose. Fair Trade certified coffee and teas are also available in many restaurants and cafes.

Chocolate: Found at most natural and fine food grocery stores, Fair Trade certified chocolate bars tend to be high quality, making it a great gift as well. You should also be able to find chips and bars for baking. Many popular brands are using it as an ingredient in products like snack bars, ice creams, and cookies.

Herbs and Spices: Fair Trade standards for herbs and spices ensure small farmers will receive a price that allows them to compete in the market, as well as a premium to invest in social and economic projects for their communities.

Clothing: When trying to find Fair Trade clothing, it is best to look online. This is a relatively new program that directly affects farmers who grow the cotton and the workers who sew the garments, offering consumers an opportunity to make a positive impact on lives. Participating brands include Good & Fair Clothing, HAE Now, prAna, and Tompkins Point Apparel.

Sugars and Sweeteners: In addition to being sold in bags for baking, Fair Trade-certified cane sugar is a common ingredient in products like ice cream, cookies, chocolate bars, and bottled beverages. Fair Trade-certified agave and honey are also starting to appear in more grocery stores. Sugar cane farmers are some of the most impoverished in the world due to fluctuating prices and difficulty accessing the U.S. market.

Produce: If you haven't switched to Fair Trade bananas, now is the time. As the most common certified fruit, bananas are now available in many grocery stores around the country. If yours doesn't carry them, be sure to make a request. You may also find Fair Trade pineapples, mangoes, cucumbers, bell peppers, peaches and more.

Stores in my community that stock Fair Trade Items:

....

....

....

....

GRATITUDE LIST

Gratitude is the fairest blossom, which springs from the soul.

— HENRY WARD BEECHER

Background

Prominent researcher, Robert Emmons, defines gratitude as, "a feeling of wonder, thankfulness, and appreciation for life." While the concept of gratitude for one's blessing is not a new one, it wasn't until the science of positive psychology emerged at the turn of the 21st century that the act of gratitude could be definitively proven as a strategy to increase happiness. How you *think* about yourself and your life, it turns out, is far more important than your actual circumstances. Gratitude keeps us focused on what we have in the present moment, which makes us happier and more hopeful. This, in turn, makes us less inclined to be anxious, lonely, depressed, envious, or neurotic.

Getting Started

It has been said that gratitude has one of the strongest links to mental health as any character trait. In addition, it's one of the easiest acts to carry out, requiring only a pen and notebook, or computer, and thoughtful countenance. There are numerous resources available online including gratitude journal templates, inspirational writings, and tips. Research shows the act of completing a gratitude list has greater impact if it is carried out one day each week rather than daily. It's important to note after creating your weekly list, you will want to reflect momentarily on each item so that it is not just a task to be completed but truly imbues you with a sense of well being and joy.

Noteworthy

- According to Sonja Lyubomirsky, who wrote *The How of Happiness*, expressing gratitude bolsters self-worth and self-esteem. The practice of gratitude encourages you to consider what you value about your current life and how much you have accomplished, making you more confident and productive.

- Gratitude helps build social bonds by strengthening existing relationships and nurturing new ones. Keeping a gratitude journal can produce feelings of greater connectedness with others by becoming aware of the value of your friends and family members.

- Gratitude helps people deal more effectively with stress and trauma, so that negative memories are less likely to surface and with less intensity in those who are regularly grateful. Expressing gratitude during times of personal adversity can help you adapt, move forward, and begin anew.

Directions: Begin the practice of counting your blessings by keeping a gratitude journal. Choose one day a week to ponder 3–5 things for which you are grateful. Don't forget to reflect on them for a moment once they are written.

WEEK 1

1.

2.

3.

4.

5.

WEEK 2

1.

2.

3.

4.

5.

WEEK 3

1.

2.

3.

4.

5.

WEEK 4

1.

2.

3.

4.

5.

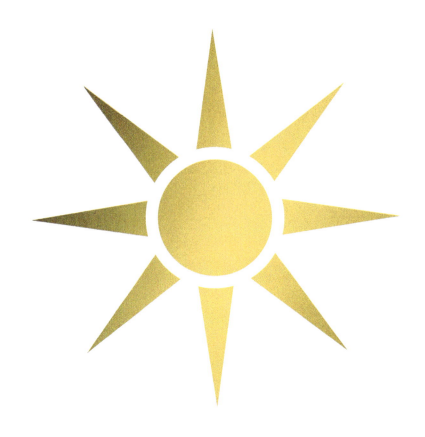

+ ENERGY

(HEALTH AND WELLNESS)

Discover the critical areas of physical well being to maximize your energy potential

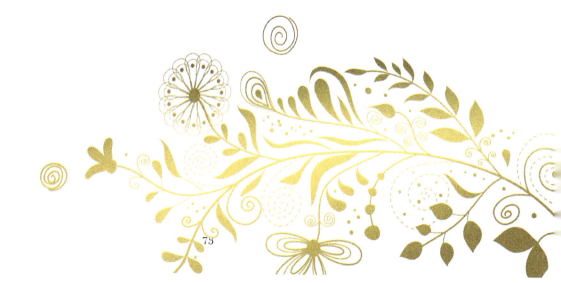

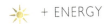

MOVING FOR ENERGY

It is exercise alone that supports the spirits, and keeps the mind in vigor.

— MARCUS TULLIUS CICERO

Background

When National Geographic explorer Dan Buettner traveled the globe to uncover the secrets of the world's six Blue Zones (concentrated areas with the greatest number of centenarians), he identified nine habits that people of longevity share. One of those is moderate, natural daily exercise. Okinawans, for instance, garden, walk, frequently practice some form of martial arts, and perform traditional Okinawan dance. The human body was meant for movement. To maintain optimal health as we age, we need to find opportunities to keep it moving.

Getting Started

It's never too late to reap the rewards of fitness. Become familiar with the four types of exercise on the following page and make a concerted effort to work them into your week if you aren't already doing so. If the idea of working out at home or in the gym leaves you underwhelmed, spend time thinking outside the box in terms of how you might exercise. Consider non-traditional exercise such as salsa dancing, ice skating, hula hoop, ultimate Frisbee, cross-country skiing, rowing, snow shoeing, or volksmarsching. Volksmarsching is a non-competitive fitness walking that originated in Europe, but includes an American counterpart called the American Volkssport Association.

Noteworthy

* Physical activity is associated with a reduced risk or slower progression of several age-related conditions, less disability, and better overall health and longevity.

* Researchers have found that chronic psychological stress appears to shorten telomeres (the protective "caps" on the end of chromosomes that indicate cell health and age), a problem associated with cardiovascular disease, cancer, and other age-related diseases. Regular physical activity may moderate the impact of stress and protect telomeres against damage.

* If even a half hour of exercise seems undoable, try fitting in two or three 10-minute sessions throughout the day to start. Studies suggest multiple shorter blocks to be as effective as longer sessions. This could amount to a quick walk around the block, dancing during commercials, jumping on a mini-tramp, or running the stairs in your house.

Directions: Design an exercise program that fits your schedule, temperament, and physical ability while trying to incorporate each of the four exercise types.

AEROBIC

Examples: Running, climbing stairs, jumping rope, cross-country skiing, aerobic or step classes, cycling, snowshoeing, dancing, swimming

Benefits: Increases stamina and conditions the heart, increases the flow of oxygen to all systems, stimulates circulation, and helps manage stress by triggering the release of endorphins.

Aim for: 30 minutes, five times a week

Keep in mind: You may wish to find a low impact aerobic class or try water aerobics.

FLEXIBILITY

Examples: Yoga, stretch classes or DVDs

Benefits: Improves your range of motion, maintains the health of tendons, ligaments, and joints, compensates for longs hours stooped over desks and computers.

Aim for: 2 to 3 days a week

Keep in mind: Yoga offers a number of benefits in and of itself. Performed regularly, it reduces chronic back pain and has a positive effect on the nervous system. It leads to deep relaxation and is a powerful stress reducer.

STRENGTH TRAINING

Examples: Lifting with weights, lunges, abdominal exercises, weight machines, bicep curls and triceps extensions, bench press or shoulder press

Benefits: Linked to better balance, lower risk of falls and fractures, better blood sugar control, reduced pain from arthritis, less depression, and improved cognitive function.

Aim for: At least 2 days a week

Keep in mind: Technique is important to avoid injury so it might be worth it to invest in a personal trainer. Allow 48 hours between sessions.

BALANCE

Examples: Some standing yoga poses, BOSU balls (available at health clubs and from online retailers), tai chi, walking on uneven ground

Benefits: Significantly reduces risk of injury from falls, promotes flexibility and good body awareness.

Aim for: 2 to 3 days a week

Keep in mind: Even standing on one leg while talking on the phone or brushing your teeth with eyes open or closed is effective for enhancing balance.

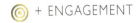

THIS I BELIEVE

Strong beliefs win strong men, and then make them stronger.

— RICHARD BACH

Background

This I Believe began as a radio program of the same name, hosted by acclaimed journalist Edward R. Murrow. Murrow said the program sought "to point to the common meeting grounds of beliefs, which is the essence of brotherhood and the floor of our civilization." Despite the difficult era of the time, which included atomic warfare, the contributors to Murrow's series expressed tremendous hope. Each day millions of Americans gathered by their radios to listen to the compelling essays of such people as Eleanor Roosevelt, Jackie Robinson, Helen Keller, and Harry Truman as well as unknown individuals in all walks of life.

The radio series became a cultural phenomenon with eighty-five leading newspapers printing a weekly column based on the series. A collection of essays was printed in 1952 and sold 300,000 copies, second only to the Bible that year. The series was revived by Dan Gediman and Jay Allison on NPR from 2005 – 2009. Since late 2010, all new *This I Believe* segments have been broadcast on *Bob Edwards Weekend*. Several subsequent books containing collections of essays have been printed since the original.

Getting Started

In the coming week determine a belief that has shaped your life in a unique or unusual way. Using the guidelines listed on the following page, capture the essence of that belief in a short 350–500 word essay. You may choose to involve other family members or close friends in this project by sharing guidelines with them, collecting the essays, and formatting them into a simply bound book. If you added a decorative cover and photo of participating members on the back cover, you would have a unique Christmas gift that would be not only inexpensive, but meaningful.

Noteworthy

- In reviving *This I Believe* in 2004, executive producer Dan Gediman said, "The goal is not to persuade Americans to agree on the same beliefs. Rather, the hope is to encourage people to begin the much more difficult task of developing respect for beliefs different from their own."

- Jay Allison added, "As in the 1950s, this is a time when belief is dividing the nation and the world. We are not listening well, not understanding each other – we are simply disagreeing, or worse. Working in broadcast communication, there's a responsibility to change that, to cross borders, to encourage some empathy. That possibility is what inspires me about this series."

Directions: Create your own *This I Believe* essay using the writing guidelines listed below.

Tell a Story: Being as specific as possible, draw upon beliefs that have been shaped by your own life experiences. What do you know that someone else might not? Don't worry about being heart-warming or gut-wrenching, you can even be funny, as long as you are genuine. Make sure your story ties to the essence of your daily life philosophy and the shaping of your beliefs.

Be Brief: Your statement should be between 350–500 words (that's about three minutes when read aloud at a natural pace.)

Name Your Belief: If you can't name it in a sentence or two, your essay may not be about a belief. Your mission is to focus on one core belief that you hold dear.

Be Positive: Avoid preaching or editorializing. Tell us what you believe, not what you don't believe. Avoid speaking in the editorial "we." Make your essay about you and speak in the first person.

Be Personal: Write in words and phrases that are comfortable for you to speak. You might want to read your essay to yourself several times, and then edit it and simplify it until you find the words, tone and story that truly echo your belief as well as the way you speak.

Brainstorm possible topic themes here (suggestions are also available online, grouped by theme):

MINDFULNESS MEDITATION

Half an hour's meditation each day is essential, except when you are busy, then a full hour is needed.
— ST. FRANCIS DE SALES

Background

Buddha believed that the source of suffering comes from trying to escape our direct experiences. We cause this suffering by attempting to move away from pain and toward pleasure. Instead of easing our suffering or increasing our happiness, however, it has the opposite effect. The second source of suffering comes from trying to assume a false identity known as the ego. The practice of mindfulness allows us to simply be with our experiences, whether pleasant , unpleasant, or neutral. When we are mindful, we show up for our own lives, rather than missing them by being distracted or wishing things were different.

Getting Started

The best way to nurture mindfulness is through sitting meditation, a practice that provides us the opportunity to be with ourselves just as we are. This, in turn, gives us glimpses of inherent wisdom and teaches us to stop perpetuating the unnecessary suffering that comes from trying to escape discomfort or even pain. This week, become familiar with the practice of mindfulness meditation by striving to sit for 10 or more minutes. If you find it difficult to sit for even that period of time, consider utilizing a guided meditation, which can be downloaded from the Internet. John Kabot-Zinn, creator of the Center for Mindfulness in Medicine, Health Care, and Society, is an excellent resource in the area of mindfulness meditation and offers a variety of guided meditations.

Noteworthy

- Meditation has been shown to increase serotonin, which influences moods and behavior. Low levels of serotonin are associated with depression and insomnia.

- In addition, meditation lowers blood pressure, reduces heart risk, and enhances the immune system by decreasing the amount of free radicals in our system. Master meditators, defined as those who meditate a minimum of twenty minutes twice a day, have been shown to live an average of seven additional years.

- Meditation shifts the mind away from worries that plague us to the present moment. We are distracted from negative thoughts that threaten our peace of mind. In addition, meditation has been shown to increase productivity and retard aging of the brain.

Directions: Bring the practice of mindfulness meditation to your week, using the following guidelines. Strive to incorporate the practice into your daily routine.

Time: If you are new to meditation, begin by sitting for 10 or 15 minutes. Gradually increase the time allotment to 20 or 30 minutes. Eventually, you may wish to sit upwards of 45 minutes. An important factor of meditation is consistency so choose the time that works best for you and strive to follow through daily.

Location: Choose an environment that is comfortable and free of distractions. This may be a corner of a room or similarly quiet space. Some individuals choose to create a small altar of some type and decorate it with pictures or sacred items that are personally significant. You may also choose to light candles or burn incense during your practice.

Posture: Sitting meditation can be done on a chair or cross-legged on the ground. Meditation pillows, called zafus or gomdens, can also be used to perch on with the legs crossed. Whether on a chair or cushion, make sure your hips are higher than your knees to avoid stress on your back. You want a posture that is upright and dignified, but not rigid. If sitting on the floor or a cushion, cross your legs comfortably in front of you with hands resting on the thighs or in your lap. You may have your eyes closed or keep them open with your gaze resting unfocused in front of you.

Practice: Once you are comfortably seated, begin to settle your attention to your breath, as you continue to breathe normally. Notice your belly as it expands on the in breath and contracts on the out breath. Or you may prefer to focus on the feel of air moving in and out of your nostrils. Each time your mind wanders away from your breath, note where it went and gently bring it back to the belly or the nostril. Remember, the purpose of mindfulness meditation is not to have any thoughts whatsoever, but to be mindful of whatever is happening as it happens. Be yourself as you are, not as some preconceived notion of what you should be.

Mindfulness Meditation Practice for the Week

SUNDAY

MONDAY

TUESDAY

WEDNESDAY

THURSDAY

FRIDAY

SATURDAY

ADDITIONAL NOTES:

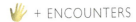

BOOKS AND BRUNCH

Books are the quietest and most constant of friends; they are the most accessible and wisest of counselors, and the most patient of teachers.

— CHARLES WILLIAM ELLIOT

Background

Nothing bolsters the spirit more than a good book or a good friend, so why not combine the two in a social event guaranteed to deliver lively conversation and deepened friendships? During the months of March or April, when many parts of the country are still damp and chilly, plan a weekend brunch with old and new friends centered around delicious food and stimulating books. This event differs from a book club, which typically meets monthly and requires all members to read the same book. During this get together participants will be asked to bring a favorite book they have read during the year to share.

Getting Started

Once a date and time have been decided upon, give your invitees plenty of time to respond and search their bookshelves. To make the occasion more notable, create a unique invitation using a bookmark. If you are making it yourself, incorporate the information right into the design of the bookmark. Or if you prefer to purchase them at a book or novelty store, print the information on the back or onto decorative paper that can then be wrapped around the bookmark. After the event they will have a small reminder of the enjoyable day together with friends.

Noteworthy

- Occasions such as Books and Brunch provide numerous benefits for participants. Not only are you receiving the positive emotions that come from socializing with others, but you also are employing creativity through the making of the invitations, the decoration of the table, and cooking of the meal. In addition, you are engaging the mind during the discussion.

- Brunches are often the forgotten opportunity in terms of entertaining, but generally easier to pull off than cocktail parties with multiple appetizers or a full sit-down dinner. There is generally less conflict with other social engagements as well, due to the early time of day.

- The idea of brunch is credited to an Englishman named Guy Beringer who in 1895 published an article in the magazine *Hunter's Weekly* titled, "Brunch: A Plea." Tired of the standard heavy English meal served right after church, Beringer pitched the idea of a lighter meal around noon with breakfast items for late risers.

Directions: During the week set a date for your own Books and Brunch using the following ideas for inspiration and motivation. If successful, you may choose to make it an annual event.

Books and Brunch

Date: Selected date

Time: Selected time

Address: Your address

Please bring a favorite book you've read this year to share with others!

RSVP: Regrets only

Phone number and email address

Menu

- Make-ahead egg casserole/quiche

- Sliced ham or bacon knots

- 2–3 types of sweetbread, scones, and muffins from bakery

- Fresh fruit salad with simple syrup dressing

The Festive Table

After setting your table with tablecloth or placemats, carry the theme of the brunch to the center of your table using two or three stacks of books alternately angled along the length. These can be used as a foundation for small containers of fresh greenery and candles. For an additional touch fill small frames with quotes by famous authors.

Have pads of paper and pens at each place so that your guests may take notes during the presentation of books.

ADDITIONAL NOTES:

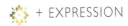

TYPES OF CREATIVE INTELLIGENCE

We have to continually be jumping off cliffs and developing our wings on the way down.
— KURT VONNEGUT

Background

In 1983 Howard Gardner introduced the theory of multiple intelligences in his book *Frames of Mind: The Theory of Multiple Intelligences*. His groundbreaking model presented the concept of intelligence as comprised of specific "modalities" rather than one single general ability. He chose eight abilities to meet his criteria including: musical/rhythmic; visual/spatial; verbal/linguistic; logical/mathematical; bodily/kinesthetic; interpersonal; intrapersonal; and naturalistic. According to Gardner, intelligence: 1) creates an effective product or offers a service of value to society; 2) makes it possible for a person to solve problems in life; 3) creates solutions for problems by gathering new information.

Getting Started

The eight multiple intelligences offer a variety of options for the individual trying to increase her personal level of creativity. Although each of us is endowed with all eight of the intelligences, we tend to rely on the same few, which we are naturally drawn to or highlight our strongest skills. In the following exercise, you will be asked to experiment with all eight categories in the coming weeks. This will require working outside your comfort zone in order to strengthen brain connections and unleash your inner creative soul.

Noteworthy

◇ What are your three strongest modalities?

1. ....

2. ....

3. ....

◇ Your three weakest modalities?

1. ....

2. ....

3. ....

Directions: Experiment with a different activity each week to help strengthen all eight of your intelligences and restore creative energy.

Musical/Rhythmic: Musical intelligence includes the capacity to discern pitch, rhythm, tone, and timbre in order to create, recognize, reproduce, and appreciate all forms of music. *Tap your musical talents by attending concerts, dusting off an old instrument, dancing to a CD with a strong beat, dragging friends to a night of karaoke, and enjoying rhythms.*

Visual/Spatial: Spatial intelligence allows you to think in 3-D through mental imagining and spatial reasoning. Architects, pilots, sailors, and sculptors are all examples of fields that rely heavily on spatial capabilities. *Flex your visual and spatial muscles through painting or drawing, create logos, map out a route, design a garden or room, play with mazes and jigsaw puzzles.*

Verbal/Linguistic: Linguistic intelligence is the ability to think in words by using language to express complex thoughts and emotions. Of all the creative intelligences, it is linguistic that is expressed most widely and proficiently by humans. *Write a weekly essay on a topic of your choice, tell stories, attend lectures, give interviews, and do a crossword puzzle.*

Logical/Mathematical: This area of creative intelligence fosters our thinking as to how numbers are incorporated into our lives in ways we don't normally consider. It deals with logic, abstractions, calculations, and hypotheses. Those individuals with well-developed logicalmathematical intelligence are interested in patterns, categories, and relationships. *Make a point to solve problems, design budgets, create schedules, and balance the checkbook.*

Bodily/Kinesthetic: This mind-body connection involves being able to manipulate objects and use a variety of physical skills. Gardner includes with this a sense of timing and the ability to train responses. *Strive to move in a variety of ways such as swimming, doing yoga, jump roping, or playing one of the options from Wii.*

Interpersonal/Social: Individuals with high interpersonal intelligence communicate effectively and empathize with others. They work to connect socially through rich, involved conversations with people of different backgrounds and cultures. *Collaborate on a project with someone who possesses different strengths than your own, invite someone from a different culture into your home, discuss ideas with a variety of acquaintances, exchange ideas, and build relationships.*

Intrapersonal: Intrapersonal intelligence, also called learned common sense, develops through self-reflection and introspection. It involves a deep capacity to understand oneself and to use that information in directing one's life. *Conquer a problem by reading a self-help book, keep a journal of daily reflection, and study the teachings of philosophers and spiritual leaders.*

Naturalistic: If you're feeling uninspired creatively, consider moving outdoors to help stir insight and connections. Nature has the unique ability to relax you, allowing new ideas to flow more easily. *Become a bird lover, garden, collect specimens, follow animal tracks, and photograph landscapes.*

CELEBRATING SENIORS

The wiser mind mourns less for what age takes away than what it leaves behind.
— WILLIAM WORDSWORTH

Background

As modern culture has become increasingly youth obsessed, individuals no longer in the work force or entirely self-reliant are often overlooked. Our perception of seniors is further skewed with stereotyped movie roles, depressing media reports, and a general unease with the aging process. Unfortunately, the result is often isolated seniors living out their final years unable to share with others their collective wisdom and life experience. By making an effort to understand the changing attributes and challenges of our society's eldest members, we can simultaneously benefit from their deep understanding of human nature while providing relief for their physical decline.

Getting Started

Our first interaction with caring for the elderly is often at home when we are called upon to accompany aging parents to doctor visits, provide help within the home or apartment, and assist in the process of finding suitable living arrangements once a parent is unable to remain at home. If your parents do not require additional care, have passed away, or do not live in close proximity, consider sharing your time and talents with other deserving seniors in your community.

Noteworthy

- Although the physical benefits of a robust social life has been clearly demonstrated, it is estimated 43 percent of seniors who live in their own home experience social isolation. Social isolation among seniors is linked to increased risk of falls, increased dementia, and increased re-hospitalization, as well as lower life expectancy.

- Numerous opportunities to interact with seniors can be found on the Internet pairing volunteers with the elderly to perform light cleaning, run errands, or provide transportation. There is even an organization that arranges monthly teas for six to eight seniors with volunteers either providing transportation or acting as host.

- If your community does not provide senior volunteer options, create your own. Consider joining with friends to bring pets to a nursing home, launch a senior walking program, start a computer lab for seniors, hold monthly seminars on nutrition, or host regular story telling hours.

Directions: Look through the following suggestions for volunteering with seniors and choose one or two to carry out in the coming weeks.

1. **Promote a sense of purpose:** Seniors should be encouraged to remain active with hobbies and interests. Those who continue to enjoy performances, participate in exercise classes, or attend community events are much better off than those who sit passively.

2. **Give a senior a pet or plant to care for:** Research indicates the act of nurturing can relieve feelings of social isolation. Pet owners suffer less depression and loneliness, giving them a reason to get up in the morning.

3. **Encourage religious seniors to continue attending their place of worship:** The weekly ritual of attending religious services is of utmost importance to many seniors. Not only do they benefit from the social connection and sense of purpose, but other worshippers help monitor their welfare.

4. **Make transportation available:** Lack of adequate transportation is a leading cause of social isolation for seniors. Helping run errands or merely taking them for a drive will promote a feeling of normalcy and independence.

5. **Encourage hearing and vision screening:** Seniors with untreated hearing or vision problems are at a disadvantage in situations where they must converse. A hearing aid may be all that is needed to improve outings.

6. **Encourage dining with others:** Sharing a meal with others is a fundamental need for all individuals and one many seniors must forgo. Whether it's eating with a neighbor, volunteering, joining in at a church potluck or senior center, it's important that seniors frequently have the option to dine with others.

7. **Give extra support to seniors who have recently lost a spouse:** Older adults are most vulnerable when they have lost a spouse, particularly one of many years. Endeavor to provide additional support to widows and widowers as others drop out of the picture.

8. **Provide support for a caregiver:** Another way to help out seniors is by providing relief for a caregiver to a senior. Studies show up to 70 percent of caregivers suffer depression due to social isolation and lack of time to care for themselves. Pitch in whenever possible to make their life easier.

What interaction, if any, do I currently have with seniors?

What opportunities for assisting seniors exist in my community?

What is my goal in this area for the coming year?

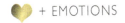

RANDOM ACTS OF KINDNESS

That best portion of a good man's life; His little, nameless, unremembered acts of kindness and love.
— WILLIAM WORDSWORTH

Background

The Random Acts of Kindness movement is credited to a woman in Sausalito, California who, in 1982, scrawled the words *Practice random acts of kindness and senseless acts of beauty* on a placemat. A quiet but steady movement grew from those words, leading to the 1993 book *Random Acts of Kindness*, which featured the true stories of such acts. Soon afterwards, a chain reaction of awareness was created with numerous articles appearing in newspapers and radios devoting airtime to the cause. Today, RAK is a well established concept, known for bringing happiness to both initiator and recipient.

Getting Started

Opportunities to practice kindness are all around us. While carrying out random acts of kindness may initially seem contrived, you will find yourself discovering multiple ways to lighten the load for someone else. A few ideas to get you started include: being extra nice to a telemarketer, leaving a note of thanks for the person who makes your coffee each morning, raking your neighbor's yard, giving blood or becoming an organ donor, being kind to someone you dislike, donating a used vehicle to a charity, praising a parent for their child, writing a short letter to the boss of an employee who went to great lengths to serve you, or putting change in a lapsed parking meter

Noteworthy - Taken from *The How of Happiness* by Sonja Lyubormirsky

- ♥ **Timing**: Research indicates when it comes to practicing kindness, doing too little negates the benefit. Consequently if you do too much, you may end up feeling resentful and burdened. A good plan would be to pick one day per week when you commit to one large act of kindness, or three to five smaller ones.

- ♥ **Variety**: Practicing the same act regularly may become less gratifying with time than alternating your choices. This appears to matter less if the commitment involves regular contact with other people (i.e. tutoring a student, taking a sick neighbor to doctor appointments, helping out with the same fundraiser).

- ♥ **Outcome**: The end result of your act of kindness may have a larger cumulative effect than you realize. The recipient is more likely to turn around and extend a similar favor to someone in their proximity, creating a "ripple effect" of compassion.

Directions: Commit one day a week to practice one large or 3–5 small RAK

Designated day of week:

Ideas for RAK:

RAK:

HAPPINESS EFFECT:

WOULD I DO AGAIN?:

RAK:

HAPPINESS EFFECT:

WOULD I DO AGAIN?:

RAK:

HAPPINESS EFFECT:

WOULD I DO AGAIN?:

RAK:

HAPPINESS EFFECT:

WOULD I DO AGAIN?:

RAK:

HAPPINESS EFFECT:

WOULD I DO AGAIN?:

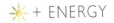

SUPPLEMENTING FOR ENERGY

A healthy outside starts from the inside.

— ROBERT URICH

Background

Keeping your body in optimum condition begins with a basic understanding of the essential vitamins and minerals your body uses for a variety of biological processes such as digestion, metabolism, and nerve function. There are 13 vitamins the body requires, including A, C, D, E, K and the B vitamins (thiamine, riboflavin, niacin, pantothenic acid, biotin, B-6, B-12, and folate.) Fat-soluble vitamins (A, D, E, K) are absorbed into the body with the use of bile acids, with the body storing for use as needed. Be cautious of over consumptionwith fat-soluble vitamins, which can lead to toxicity. Water-soluble vitamins (all the remaining) are easily absorbed by the body, with the kidneys removing those not needed.

Getting Started

Develop a personal vitamin strategy, keeping in mind that food sources are always the best option for vitamins and minerals. Consume a variety of nutrient-dense food from all major food groups, limiting the intake of saturated and trans fats, cholesterol, added sugars, salt, and alcohol. The purpose of supplements is to fill a nutrient gap that cannot or is not being met by the intake of food. Do not take the addition of supplements lightly, as there is a risk of over doing it, particularly with fat-soluble vitamins.

Noteworthy

* There are a few supplements nearly everyone can benefit from, including a quality multivitamin, vitamin D (especially if you live in a sun-deprived state), an omega-3 boost like fish or flax oil, vitamin B12 if you are vegan, and calcium. You're better off getting antioxidants from bright, fresh fruits and vegetables.

* Look for vitamins in easily absorbed capsule form with enteric coating versus harder-to-digest tablet versions. Skip liquid supplements, which may be easier to swallow but often deficient in enzymes that aid in vitamin absorption.

* Some nutritionists recommend taking an organic multivitamin like New Chapter, Blue Bonnet, or Solgar rather than drugstore brands as they are absorbed more readily and you don't end up over-dosing or excreting excess.

* Many fat-soluble vitamins are stored in the body for up to 24 hours, making it important to take them at roughly the same time each day. If you are taking other medications, be sure you ask your doctor whether they interact with vitamins. Calcium, for instance, interferes with the absorption of levothyroxine for hypothyroidism and must be taken at a different time.

Directions: Develop a supplemental strategy, bearing in mind your age, eating habits, and health needs. Discuss the strategy, including proper dosage with your physician before initiating.

Vitamin A: Essential for vision, keeps tissues and skin healthy, important for bone growth, may lower risk of lung cancer and cataracts. (Beef, liver, eggs, shrimp, fish, fortified milk, cheddar and Swiss cheese)

Vitamin B6: May reduce heart disease, helps make red blood cells and influences cognitive abilities and immune function. (Meat, fish, poultry, legumes, tofu and other soy products, potatoes, non-citrus fruits such as bananas and watermelon)

Vitamin B12: Assists in making new cells and breaking down some fatty acids and amino acids, protects nerve cells and encourages their normal growth. (Meat, poultry, fish, milk, cheese, eggs, fortified cereals)

Vitamin C: May lower the risk of some cancers and cataracts, helps make collagen and the neurotransmitter serotonin, acts as an antioxidant and bolsters immune system. (Fruit and fruit juices, potatoes, broccoli, bell peppers, spinach, strawberries, tomatoes, Brussels sprouts)

Vitamin D: Helps form teeth and bones, and supplements can reduce number of non-spinal fractures. Many people don't get enough of this nutrient, particularly if you live in a northern climate or don't spend much time in the sun. (Fortified milk or margarine, fortified cereals, fatty fish)

Vitamin E: Acts as an antioxidant, neutralizing unstable molecules that can damage cells, diets rich in vitamin E may help protect against Alzheimer's. (Vegetable oils, salad dressings, wheat germ, leafy green vegetables, whole grains, nuts)

Calcium: Builds bones and teeth, helps with blood clotting and nerve impulse transmission, plays a role in hormone secretion and enzyme activation, helps maintain healthy blood pressure. (Yogurt, cheese, milk, sardines, salmon, fortified juices, broccoli, kale)

Iron: Helps hemoglobin in red blood cells, needed for chemical reactions in the body and for making amino acids, collagen, and hormones. (Red meat, poultry, eggs, fruits, green vegetables, fortified bread, and grain products)

Magnesium: Needed for many chemical reactions in the body, works with calcium in muscle contraction, blood clotting, and regulation of blood pressure. (Green vegetables such as spinach and broccoli, legumes, cashews, seeds, halibut, whole wheat bread, milk)

Selenium: Acts as an antioxidant, neutralizing unstable molecules that damage cells, helps regulate thyroid hormone activity. (Organ meats, seafood, walnuts, grain products)

Zinc: Needed for immune system, taste, smell, and wound healing, may help delay the progression of age-related macular degeneration. (Red meat, poultry, oysters, and some seafood, fortified cereals, beans, nuts)

ADDITIONAL NOTES:

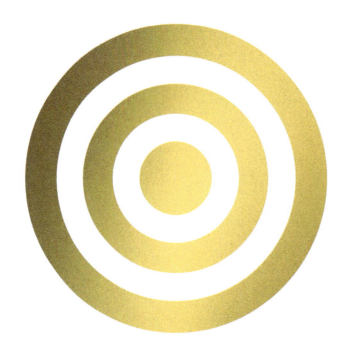

+ ENGAGEMENT

(INTELLECTUAL STIMULATION)

Study the upside of meaningful engagement
and the powerful concept of "flow"

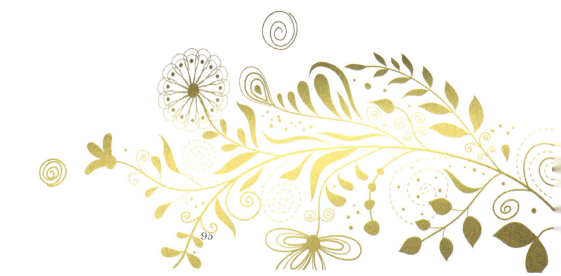

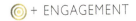

LEARNING INSPIRATION BOARD

The love of learning, the sequestered nooks,
And all the sweet serenity of books.

— HENRY WADSWORTH LONGFELLOW

Background

Up until recently, scientists believed the brain reached full maturity very early in life and once fully formed, the wiring of the brain as well as nerve cells (neurons) were immutable. That viewpoint meant an individual was stuck with the brain they were born with and little, if anything, could be done to alter this fact. It also meant statistically for those people who reached their 85th birthday, roughly half would experience cognitive decline in the form of dementia or Alzheimer's. Through the emerging science of brain-plasticity we now know we are not, in fact, hardwired from birth. In truth, the brain possesses an astonishing ability to remodel itself through the acquisition and refinement of new skills and abilities. This means it is never too late to sustain and even bypass current levels of brain function.

Getting Started

Continuing to acquire new information and skills throughout the span of our lifetime is imperative to maintaining a healthy and pliable brain well into old age. Make this goal a priority by devoting a small area of your environment toward its endeavor. To begin, start gathering ideas for areas of study — magazine articles of interest, current schedules of community/university classes, times and locations of local museums, TED talk topics you'd like to explore, and additional academic resources that are available where you live. Once affixed to some type of surface, this tool will help remind and inspire you to meet your ongoing learning goals.

Noteworthy

- TED talks (Technology/Entertainment/Design) can be accessed online free of charge and provide an endless source of thought-provoking ideas to challenge your brain. Take your learning even farther by writing down your thoughts on a specific talk or waiting a couple days to record everything you remember about it.

- Once you have your inspiration board complete, don't forget to include evidence of learning goals met throughout the year such as ticket stubs to a speaker or conference, check marks next to museums visited, and scores for items memorized.

Directions: Using a bulletin board, large foam board, or back wall of a computer station begin accumulating topics of learning that will motivate you and provide multiple opportunities for exploration throughout the year.

TOPICS OF INTEREST

1.
2.
3.
4.
5.
6.
7.
8.

DON'T FORGET:

History Museums
Art Museums
Local Points of Interest
Art Galleries
Cultural Landmarks
Botanical Gardens
Historical Homes
Landmark depots
Train Stations
Prisons

COMMUNITY/UNIVERSITY CLASSES

1.

2.

3.

4.

TED TALKS

TOPIC / SPEAKER:

TOPIC / SPEAKER:

TOPIC / SPEAKER:

TOPIC / SPEAKER:

ADDITIONAL NOTES:

LETTER OF FORGIVENESS

When you hold resentment toward another, you are bound to that person or condition by an emotional link that is stronger than steel. Forgiveness is the only way to dissolve that link and get free.

— CATHERINE PONDER

Background

Since 1990, Dr. Everett Worthington, a psychology professor at Virginia Commonwealth University, had been a leading researcher on forgiveness, counseling Holocaust and Rwanda's genocide victims. On New Year's morning in 1996, he received a call from his brother telling him his mother had been murdered – brutally raped before being bludgeoned to death with a crowbar. The successful struggle of Dr. Washington to forgive the individuals responsible has been an inspiration to many. His 5-step plan of forgiveness is called REACH:

Recall: Recall the hurtful events as accurately and objectively as possible.

Empathize: Try to understand what happened from the viewpoint of the person who wronged you.

Altruistic gift of forgiveness: Recall a time you hurt someone else and were forgiven. Offer this gift to the person who wronged you.

Commit yourself to forgive publicly: Write a letter of forgiveness (whether or not you send it), tell a trusted friend, write in a journal, or tell the person directly.

Holding onto forgiveness: Forgiving is not forgetting. Remind yourself you made a choice to forgive when memories arise.

Getting Started

Grievances begin when something happens in our life we don't want to happen and we begin spending an inordinate amount of time thinking about it. To avoid becoming ongoing victims, consider writing a letter of forgiveness to a person who has wronged you. You may ultimately wish to send the letter, but often such letters are written without the intent of sending but instead as an exercise in letting go of anger.

Noteworthy

- People who blame other people for their troubles have higher incidences of illnesses such as cardiovascular disease and cancers. It may be more significant than hostility as a risk factor for heart disease. People who are able to forgive their offender report immediate improvement in their cardiovascular, muscular, and nervous systems.

- Each time you read a story of forgiveness in a newspaper or magazine, clip it and store it in a file. Reminding yourself of the struggles others have overcome to forgive will inspire you to do the same.

Directions: Using the following template, compose your letter of forgiveness. If you are contemplating sending the letter, share the letter with someone you trust and get feedback. If it feels right, send the letter.

1. **Accept responsibility -** Start by accepting responsibility for the relationship with the person to whom you're writing the letter. Don't victimize yourself or blame the person for getting you into the situation you are currently.

2. **Be vulnerable -** Reveal your sadness and remorse at what transpired between you both.

3. **Forgive them for what they've done -** This is the heart of the letter. List what they've done that you are forgiving them for without being sarcastic or vengeful.

4. **State your purpose -** Let them know you are not asking them to respond in any way. You are doing this for yourself, not to be forgiven by them. If they write back, it needs to be their own choice.

5. **Positive conclusion -** If you can, include some appreciation for the person. Look at all of who they are rather than the painful interaction with you. End the letter on a positive note and wish them well by expressing hope in the future.

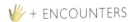

THE ART OF FRIENDSHIP

There are no strangers here; only friends you haven't yet met.

— WILLIAM BUTLER YEATS

Background

Strong social connections in the form of good friendships improve all areas of our life by providing comfort, strengthening our immune system, and warding off loneliness and depression. Meeting new friends becomes both easier and more difficult as we age. On the one hand we typically have more time and financial resources, are more self-assured with lots of different interests, and more tolerant of a variety of people. On the other hand, opportunities for making new contacts may become less obvious as our kids graduate from school, our careers begin to wind down or end, or we retire to new areas.

Getting Started

Regardless of your age, the benefits of rich and healthy friendships should remain a lifelong endeavor worthy of our effort. This is especially true if you are new to an area, recently separated or divorced, retired or changing jobs, or empty nesters. Above all, making friends requires persistency and being proactive. Make this important area of life a priority by setting goals for meeting new people and acquiring friendships.

Noteworthy

- **Where to meet friends**: Opportunities for making friends arise while volunteering for community boards and organizations; taking a class or joining a club (fitness class, book club, sports team); attending gallery openings, lectures, readings, and recitals; connecting with an alumni association; and organizing a neighborhood barbeque or dinner club.

- **How to engage in conversation**: Initiate conversation by remarking on the surroundings or event; noting something you have in common; bringing up an event in the news; complimenting the clothes or hair of the individual; sharing some self-deprecating humor; asking about books or movies they've recently seen.

- **How to be a good friend**: Don't set too many rules and expectations. You're both unique so the friendship probably will not evolve exactly as you expect. Be forgiving so that when a small issue arises you are able to overcome it; invest in the friendship by being attentive and committing regular time to help it flourish. Finally, be the friend you would like to have by being reliable, thoughtful, trustworthy, and supportive.

Directions: Practice your social connection skills by checking off each item from the checklist in the weeks ahead.

_____ I was personable and outgoing with people I met today.

_____ I've come up with a simple introduction when meeting a new person that reflects general information about myself.

_____ I've explored different retail and specialty stores in my town, introducing myself to the people who work there.

_____ I've gotten to know at least two people in my neighborhood.

_____ I regularly go where people gather.

_____ I'm consciously trying to be a good listener.

_____ I had a conversation with someone entirely different from me (in terms of looks, culture, lifestyle, etc.).

_____ My discomfort at meeting new people has lessened.

_____ I'm better at verbalizing compliments to individuals I meet.

_____ I've volunteered for a community charity or organization.

_____ I made the first move to speak to someone else new and extended a social invitation.

_____ I'm enriching my life with a new class, seminar, or lecture.

_____ I'm getting to know my coworkers (or individuals in my church, neighborhood, or association) better

_____ I hosted a social get together at my home.

_____ I initiated a conversation that resulted in a new contact or social activity.

_____ I joined a club, sports team, alumni group, or service organization

_____ I extended a spontaneous invitation for coffee, lunch, or glass of wine.

_____ I made a point of talking with my _____ (mail carrier, waiter, dry cleaner, coffee shop attendant, grocery clerk).

_____ I brought up an interesting fact from the news or radio during conversation with a new acquaintance.

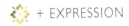

MIND MAPPING

Don't think. Thinking is the enemy of creativity. It's self-conscious, and anything self-conscious is lousy. You can't try to do things. You simply must do things.

— RAY BRADBURY

Background

Educator Tony Buzan developed the concept of Mind Mapping in the 1960s. Mind Mapping is a creative tool used to solve problems by visually connecting thoughts, ideas, and facts as the mind works. Mind maps are appropriate for creative problem solving, decision-making, project planning, brainstorming, and taking notes. At its core a mind map is a diagram that includes the arranging of words, ideas and activities linked to a central idea. The goal is to organize and classify information visually to quickly identify and understand the structure of a topic as well as how all the pieces fit together. It is similar to brainstorming, but allows for branching ideas and visually perceiving how the ideas are linked.

Getting Started

Think of a question or problem you have been struggling with and make it your focus with mind mapping. If you've wanted to improve your general overall health, start with the word Fitness in the center of your page. From there, draw curvy branches from it with related thoughts. Draw more branches from the initial ones. Mind mapping is often carried out using different colors for each major train of thought. Draw simple picture icons at the end of major branches to provide instant recall. There are a number of websites online that provide mind mapping tools.

Noteworthy

❖ Sample mind map using the concept of expanded joy.

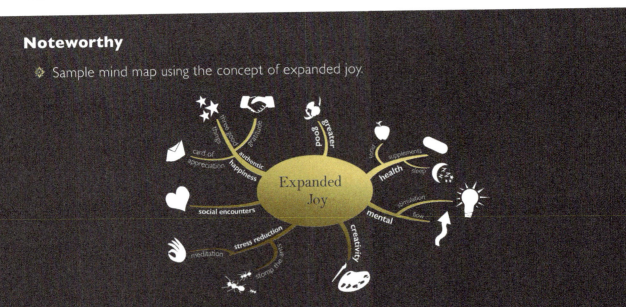

Directions: Think of a problem or project you'd like to give some thought to and write it in the center circle. Draw different color branches to brainstorm ideas, both big and small. Have fun finishing the map with simple pictures to represent each major thread of thought.

CHARITY POTLUCK

There is no exercise better for the heart than reaching down and lifting people up.

— JOHN HOLMES

Background

In 2002 Marsha Wallace gathered together for dinner a small group of twenty close friends and raised $700 throughout the evening. That dinner would eventually evolve into the national charitable organization known as *Dining For Women*. Today, in hundreds of chapters all across America, women gather together once a month, bringing a dish to share and saving their "dining out" dollars for charity. Those donations are combined to support one carefully selected international program monthly and include grass-roots programs in education, healthcare, vocational training, micro-credit loans, and economic development. The programs are aimed to improve the living situations for women and their families by providing the tools needed for change.

Getting Started

If you do not have access to a *Dining For Women* chapter or prefer to share the experience with personal friends, why not organize your own charity potluck in the comfort of your home? Potlucks remain popular due to their simplicity and convenience. With the most difficult part of entertaining – the food – taken care of, you'll find the common potluck the perfect solution to having guests to your home. Depending on the desire of the group, you may wish to make this a monthly, quarterly, or annual event.

Noteworthy

- You may choose to select a theme for your potluck such as Tex-Mex, Soup and Salad, Italian, brunch, or Potato Bar. Or, you may choose to keep it basic with people bringing a variety of dishes ranging from appetizers to dessert.

- This activity is particularly powerful, providing a double whammy of advantages. Not only will you gain the positive feelings related to the altruistic act of helping others, you also benefit from the social connection of close friends.

- If you have friends who are truly kitchen phobic, assign them something that can be purchased such as rolls, drinks, dressings, or cheese. To limit last-minute preparation, try to have guests bring their food ready to serve.

Directions: Use the following guidelines to host a charity potluck in your home at some point in the near future.

1. *Three weeks prior:* Mail or email invitations to selected friends with pertinent information including date, time, and guidelines for bringing dishes. You may wish to assign types of food (appetizer, salads, main dish, desserts) to individuals to avoid a shortage in a particular area. Be sure to let them know the purpose of the potluck (aside from seeing one another) is to raise money for a selected charity with a donation taken up at some point during the evening.

2. *Two weeks prior:* Selecting a charity can be handled a couple of ways. As the host, you can determine a charity from a local, national, or international organization. This would require some research in order to provide participants with a short program outlining the organization's mission, outreach goals, and success to date. Or, you can involve the entire group by asking each person to come with a designated charity of their choice, including relevant information to share, and have the group, after hearing the presentations, vote for their favorite.

3. *One week prior:* Secure the number who will be attending and share that information with others so that they have an idea of how much food to bring.

4. *One day prior:* Set up your buffet table or kitchen island with colorful napkins, flatware, dishes, and several serving utensils. Make sure you have places for guests to eat once they have their food. This may require card tables or small trays if not seated at a table.

5. *Day of:* Prepare food dish and set up beverage station, complete with plenty of ice. Have available notepads and pens so guests can take notes during program portion of the evening. Once guests arrive, add their dish to the designated area, ensuring there is a serving utensil available for each dish. Allow plenty of time for visiting before instructing your guests on how to proceed with the meal. Following dinner, you may need to rearrange chairs so that everyone is able to participate in the discussion.

6. *One or two days following:* Write each guest a thank you and share the amount raised for the charity. If everyone seemed to enjoy herself, you might get a feel for whether they would like to continue the event on a regular basis, rotating houses and charities.

ADDITIONAL NOTES FOR YOUR EVENT:

_____

_____

_____

_____

_____

_____

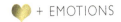

SNAP TO THE PRESENT

There is only now. And look! How rich we are in it.

— VANNA BONTA

Background

The concept of being wholly present, living in whatever moment you happen to be in as fully as possible, dates back centuries to mankind's earliest spiritual leaders. In recent years, Eckhart Tolle has perhaps become the most widely recognized expert in this area with his influential books *The Power of Now* and *A New Earth*. From writings such as Tolle's, we know there are only three possible time frames —past, present, and future. Mentally, we too often reside in the past or the future, neither of which are in our power to affect.

Getting Started

Being present might appear on the surface to be the easiest thing in the world to accomplish, but it is uniquely challenging. Begin by noticing when you are trying to change the present moment in some way and instead allow the moment to simply happen without judgment, anger, or anxiety. Rather than worrying about making your next plane connection while traveling, stay focused on what is happening around you at that moment. One way to remind yourself to stay in the moment is to wear a rubber band on your wrist. When you find your mind wandering away from what's directly in front of you, snap it gently. This simple technique will become a physical reminder of where you need to be until being present becomes habitual.

Noteworthy

- Being present strengthens **social skills**. You will find yourself listening intently to what the other person is saying rather than mentally constructing what you will say next. You should find yourself becoming less shy or awkward. Instead of feeling self-conscious, your energy is put into just being there.

- Being present makes you more **joyful**. We often are weighed down with oppressive thoughts always present in our heads. Once you let them go, you may find yourself feeling ages younger, intrigued with the beauty of each day in the same manner as a child.

- Being present makes you **calmer**. Focusing on your breathing rather than racing thoughts slows your heart rate and stills the body. The natural result is a feeling of relaxation and calmness. Strive to remind yourself of this when you begin feeling rushed or anxious.

- Being present makes you more **compassionate**. Shifting your focus to objective observations leaves little room for labeling or judging others. You don't worry about whether you or they measure up to some subjective concept in your head.

Directions: Commit to being more present in the coming week through the following practices. Make notes on when/where you tried each strategy and how you felt afterwards.

1. **Smile upon waking**: Remind yourself you are in control of your attitude each and every morning. Attract good things the day has to offer by greeting the world with a smile.

2. **Focus on what you're doing**: Whether sweeping the floor or walking the dog, relinquish extraneous thoughts racing through your head and really focus on what you are doing.

3. **Notice the world around you**: Rather than moving about on autopilot, use your senses to take note of your environment- the beauty of cut flowers, the aroma of pot roast, the sound of chimes.

4. **Minimize activities that dull your awareness**: Reduce TV watching or web surfing, both of which are passive activities. Instead, turn on music and dance. Revel in the splendors of the day!

5. **Be thankful for what you have today**: Wishing for something other than what you have keeps you from appreciating the blessings currently in your life. Don't make comparisons with others.

6. **Do one thing at a time**: Rushing is counter productive to mindfulness. Rather than multi-tasking, concentrate on doing your tasks well. Perform your tasks throughout the day with greater purpose.

7. **Stop being angry or anxious**: If you are angry, you are swept up in the past. If you are anxious, you are worried about the future. Take a moment to breathe deeply and return to the present.

ADDITIONAL NOTES:

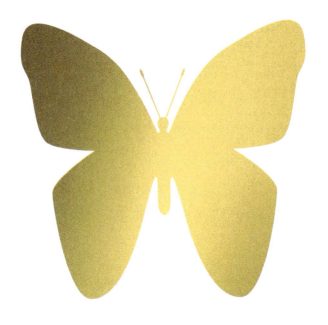

+ EASE

(INTENTIONAL CALM)

*Deflect daily stress with strategies
designed to promote genuine
serenity and well-being*

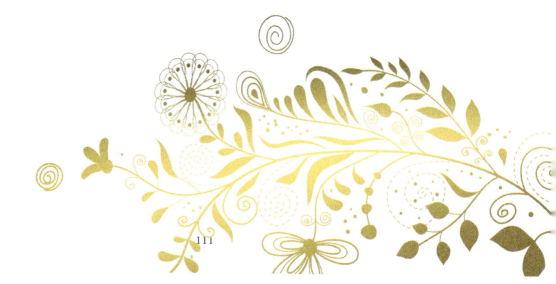

UNPLUG FOR ENERGY

My mind is constantly going. For me to completely relax, I gotta get rid of my cell phone.
— KENNY CHESNEY

Background

If you find your energy level lagging, you may want to consider whether your technology is to blame. From the automobile to the television to the computer, all technology possesses the potential to impact our life both positively and negatively. Undesirable side effects of too much time on our electronic devices include: poor sleep habits, shortened attention spans, depression, obesity, neck and back pain, constant distraction, tendonitis, and comparison living. In this modern era it would be nearly impossible not to have any interaction with technology, but we need to be cognizant of how and when we are engaged with this absorbing tool throughout the day. The goal is to achieve balance between technology use and time away from our electronics.

Getting Started

The average adult over eighteen spends nearly 11 hours a day engaged in some type of electronic media including television, smart phones, DVDs/Blue Ray, Internet, radio, and multimedia devices. Unfortunately, nearly all interaction with technology (with the exception of walking while listening to an iPod) involves sedentary behavior on the part of the user. We are sitting for unbelievably long periods, often while displaying poor posture, in front of computers, televisions, phones, e-readers, and tablets. The result of such pervasive use is frequently increased fatigue and decreased energy. In the coming week, look at your technology use to determine where you can make healthy changes.

Noteworthy

* A CNN article reported that by the time an American child reaches two, 90 percent have an online history. By age five, more than 50 percent interact regularly on the computer. The average teen texts nearly 3,500 times a month, and by middle school kids are spending more time with media than parents or teachers.

* Because light from TV and computers screens affects melatonin production, throwing off our circadian rhythm, late-night computer use has been associated with sleep disorders, stress, and depressive symptoms in both men and women. Using technology without breaks further increases the risk of stress, sleeping problems and depressive symptoms in women. A combination of heavy computer use and heavy mobile use makes the association with these symptoms even stronger.

Directions: Review the following guidelines to establish healthy technology practices and increase your energy.

1. Treat all technology equally: Whether it comes from the television, smart phone, computer, or tablet, all screen time should be treated the same. Know how much time you are spending in front of any screen throughout a typical day and strive to keep it in check.

   Total # of hours I'm spending daily with some form of technology: ....

   How can I cut back my screen time, swapping out sedentary behavior throughout the day for healthier activities? (Think small incremental steps.)

   ....
   ....
   ....
   ....
   ....
   ....
   ....

2. Be present: Regardless of what you are doing, try to be engaged to the fullest extent possible. This goes for having coffee with a friend, running errands, or hanging out with your child. Don't automatically reach for your handheld device or use it indiscriminately. Technology is meant to enhance our life, not replace it.

   When am I using technology because I'm bored or don't want to make the effort to do something more productive? (Look for patterns.)

   ....
   ....
   ....
   ....
   ....
   ....
   ....
   ....

3. Spend less time on Facebook and more time face-to-face: While social media claims connection benefits, it does not compare with actual personal contact. Being among supportive friends or close family members ranks first for boosting our feel good sensors and staving off depression.

Do I have multiple social encounters with others built into my weekly routine or am I spending more time viewing someone else's social events rather than initiating my own? If so, what steps can I take to reverse this situation?

....

....

....

....

....

....

....

4. Establish an electronic curfew: Make sure you are unplugged from all technology at least an hour prior to nodding off. Use that time to prepare mentally and physically for slumber with activities like a warm bath, stretching, having a cup of herbal tea, and reading.

My electronic curfew is:

....

....

ADDITIONAL NOTES:

....

....

....

....

....

....

ADDITIONAL NOTES:

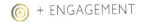

THE BEAUTIFUL BRAIN II

Great minds discuss ideas; average minds discuss events; small minds discuss people.
— ELEANOR ROOSEVELT

Background

More than five million Americans have Alzheimer's disease, the most common form of dementia, and that number is expected to triple by 2050, according to the Alzheimer's Association. Intellectual enrichment pursued over a lifetime may help reduce the number of people who will eventually come to develop the disease. David Knopman, a professor of neurology at the Mayo Clinic in Rochester, Minnesota, has stated, "Keeping your brain mentally stimulated is a lifelong enterprise. If one can remain intellectually active and stimulated throughout one's lifespan, that's protection against late-life dementia. Staying mentally active is definitely good for your brain."

Getting Started

Being aware of known deterrents to dementia is the first step in making improvements to your brain's capacity, particularly in later years. Although some of our brain's function is genetically predetermined, there is still much you can do to make the most of what you've been given. Look over the suggested activities on the following page, and make a concerted effort to incorporate as many of them as possible into your daily routine in order to maintain a beautiful brain.

Noteworthy

- As with physical exercise, exercising the brain is not something you do one time. Set a goal to perform activities that benefit your brain daily to receive maximum benefit. Factors such as diet, sleep quality, and ongoing exercise are as important to brain function as to the rest of our body.

- Something as simple as learning new words from a word-a-day calendar can enrich brain activity. Increasing your vocabulary exercises the language portion of your brain. Better yet, strive to write more frequently via a journal, blog, essay, or short story. Writing requires multiple brain functions, tapping into unused reserves.

- Most people are aware of the benefits of games such as crossword puzzles and Sudoku. But in terms of working the brain, few games are able to surpass chess. This is because it is incredibly strategic as well as tactical. Both simple to learn and easy to play, chess is the perfect hobby for anyone.

Directions: Incorporate as many of these activities as possible into your week.

1. Higher education is a known deterrent to degenerative brain diseases and a rich at-home reading program beneficial in numerous ways. Reading stimulates thought, introduces new vocabulary, and connects individuals to new ideas. To affect the brain positively, material should be both stimulating and challenging. For book ideas consider *The New York Times* "Best of the Year" list (fiction and nonfiction), which comes out each December as well as substantive magazines such as *National Geographic*, *The Smithsonian*, *The Atlantic*, *The New Yorker*, *Wired*, and *Popular Science*.

2. Another well-established deterrent to ailments of the brain is exercise, particularly the kind of exercise that leaves you breathless. Exercise has been shown to stimulate brain cell growth through a process called neurogenesis, flooding the brain with pleasurable neurotransmitters like dopamine. Most people don't realize how powerful an effect rigorous exercise can have on decreasing stress and improving cognitive performance. It is among the easiest and cheapest ways to aid in the function of your brain.

3. Diet and supplements should also be considered when looking at maximizing your mental capabilities. Researchers have found that diet can influence your brain's potential, and individuals who eat a lot of processed food tend to have lower IQs even when other factors are taken into consideration. Strive to become informed on current research regarding the impact of gluten and sugar on the brain and the importance of healthy fats and vegetables in the diet. In addition, intermittent fasting has been shown to increase the amount of Brain-Derived Neurotropic Factor (BDNF), which affects both learning and memorization. Supplements such as caffeine, fish oils, B-complex vitamins, coenzyme Q10, and magnesium have also been shown to be beneficial.

4. Meditation positively affects stress levels and mood enhancers. Additionally, it increases performance on intelligence-related measures and increases IQ over time. There are a number of different types of meditation practices, but nearly all types should improve general brain function and cognition. Generally, meditation involves sitting quietly for 10–30 minutes and focusing on your breath or a specific mantra. The practice of gently letting go of random thoughts and continually coming back to the breath or mantra, helps your brain focus on one specific thing at a time to improve overall concentration.

5. Finally, work to maintain a rich environment in your work and home space by participating in active learning and new experiences. Through active learning you can acquire new skills such as chess, foreign language, sports, or juggling. Likewise new experiences like traveling to a new location, exploring cultural opportunities, and even trying new foods help keep the brain from operating on default with the same day-to-day routines.

BOOKENDING YOUR DAY

Go in the direction of where your peace is coming from.

— C. JOYBELL

Background

How readily we handle stress throughout the day or drift off at night is greatly influenced by how we begin and end each day. And yet we often engage in activities upon waking or retiring to bed that impede our efforts of increased serenity. We live in a world that promotes 24-hour stimulation and we willingly oblige by moving through the day reading email, catching up on the latest news, monitoring a variety of social media, and passively watching TV. When we assault our senses with such activities, particularly at the beginning and end of each day, it has the negative effect of keeping us over stimulated and under inspired in a way that is neither helpful or healthy.

Getting Started

Determine how much time you can devote to a morning/evening ritual to enhance your serenity and well-being. This can be as little as 15 minutes or upwards of an hour or longer. From there, begin compiling a list of soothing activities using the menu of options on the following page or creating your own. Lastly, decide what order to carry out the selected actions to suit your needs.

Noteworthy

- If it is difficult to find time for yourself in the morning due to the schedule of other family members, consider rising a little earlier. It will be worth it in the long run if your happy countenance is transferred to those around you.

- Be particularly cognizant of when you are accessing daily news. The ratio of positive to negative news coverage is typically 10 percent to 90 percent. Be cautious of how you take in this onslaught of negative information, particularly those media outlets that intentionally format their programs to stir up feelings of anger and injustice. Commit to being informed of major news stories without becoming mired in every sordid sensation that hits the stands.

- Promote healthy rising and retiring rituals in your children or grandchildren by being mindful of how they spend the first and last minutes of their day. Soothing music, a warm bath, scented lotion, quiet reading, and a listing of what they are grateful for or their favorite part of the day will help them prepare for the day or slumber with ease.

Directions: Select from the menu of options or choose your own to create a morning and evening ritual that is meaningful.

A.M.

Hot water, splash of lemon juice

Scented candle

Deep breathing exercises

Inspirational reading

Bolt of Joy

Stretching/Yoga

Personal card to friend or family member

Crossword puzzle

Warm shower/cool rinse for energy

Oil massage

Guided meditation

Prayer of reflection

P.M.

Chamomile tea, drizzle of honey

Lavender oil

Deep breathing exercises

Educational reading

Three Good Things

Stretching/Tai chi

Journaling

To-do list

Bath/hot tub for relaxation

Foot rub

Guided relaxation exercises

Prayer of gratitude

YOUR A.M. RITUAL

YOUR P.M. RITUAL

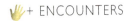

SUMMERTIME HIGH TEA

There are few hours in my life more agreeable than the hour dedicated to the ceremony known as afternoon tea.

— HENRY JAMES

Background

Tea was first discovered in China with one account dating it to the Emperor of China in 2737 B.C. During the Han Dynasty (202 B.C. – 220 AD) it was reserved for royalty due to limited tea plants and consumed for its herbal qualitites. As more tea plants were discovered in the Tang Dynasty (618 – 907), it became more common among the lower classes. It was also during this time that it spread to Japan, arriving in England during the 17th Century when King Charles II married a Portuguese princess, Catherine of Braganza. Tea soon became a popular import to Britain by way of the East India Company and afternoon tea parties became a common way for the aristocratic society to drink tea.

Getting Started

An afternoon of high tea is a fun way to connect with old friends or make new ones and certain to be a hit with your guests in a refreshing, relaxed atmosphere. There are numerous resources available online, at local teashops, or in bookstores to assist you in this endeavor. Late spring or early summer makes a perfect time of year for a tea party with temperate weather for outdoor dining and the added bonus of blooming flora. Whether set indoors or out, a pretty table that includes linens and flowers is a must. If you don't feel comfortable with the varied menu, use a reputable bakery for your scones and sweets so you have only to assemble a small assortment of finger sandwiches.

Noteworthy

- The three-tier plate holder known as the tower is traditionally stacked with scones on the top tier (jam and cream to the side), sandwiches and pastries on the second tier, and sweets on the bottom. This is also the order you eat them, even if the tower is not set according to custom.

- Tea should first be poured through a strainer into your cup with milk and sugar added later as needed. Never blow on your tea to cool it down. Two cubes or spoons of sugar are the most that is appropriate to add, stirring counter clockwise and placing the spoon on the saucer when finished.

- The correct way to signal the end of your meal is to place your knife and fork, or dessert spoon and fork, in the six o'clock position with fork tines facing up.

Directions: Think about hosting an afternoon tea for friends, young or old, using the following tips and suggestions.

TEAS

- Be sure to try a variety of teas including Earl Grey, English Breakfast, Green Tea, and herbal.
- If brewing your own, allow one scoop of dried leaves per cup and steep 2–5 minutes.
- You also may choose to simply by heating hot water in a teapot and allowing guests to choose from a selection of bagged teas.
- Remember to provide a selection of items to add to the tea including sugar, cream, lemon, and honey.

TABLE

- Choose a beautiful tablecloth aof white linen or chintz, use cloth napkins.
- Include a large tray for the tea (have coffee avaiable as well).
- Use china or porcelain dishware if possible and provide fork, butter knife, spoon, and teaspoon.
- Use a three-tiered tower for food.
- Add a small floral arrangement in center of table.

FOOD

Scones: All scones (including plain) are delicious with numerous recipes for variations using ginger, blueberries, currants, etc. Serve warm with cream and jam, and avoid freezing if possible.

Finger Sandwiches: Make fillings ahead of time and assemble shortly before party to avoid soggy bread. Use both white and wheat bread, trimming crust. Stuff with variety of fillings including egg/chicken salad, goat cheese/walnuts/red pepper, or cream cheese/smoked salmon/cucumber.

Sweets: Again, provide a variety of sweets from choolates to delicate cakes to small glasses of mousse. Work with your favorite bakery for assistance.

ADDITIONAL NOTES:

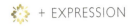

JOURNALING AND THE CURIOUS MIND

The important thing is not to stop questioning. Curiosity has its own reason for existing.
— ALBERT EINSTEIN

Background

Creative people are always on the lookout for new ideas, better solutions, fresh ways of looking at things, and stimulating experiences. Instead of spending mental energy being frustrated when they come up against something annoying or difficult, creative people use the opportunity to consider how it could be changed or altered to produce a better outcome. This way of perceiving the world comes from being intentionally more aware as you go about your day, pushing yourself to see things differently and being open to unexpected opportunities. The result is an expansion of thinking that allows you to live more fully.

Getting Started

Journaling is an excellent way to encourage the mind to think more creatively. In this particular instance a journal is not used in the same way as a diary or to simply record your activities throughout the day. Rather the journal is used to keep track of things that catch your interest, ideas that come to you while driving to work or in the shower, solutions and inventions for obstacles you are confronted with, and brainstorming lists for a new project at work. Begin a creativity journal in the coming week using the suggestions on the following page. If you commit to writing in it regularly, you will find your thoughts and ideas begin to flow more freely.

Noteworthy

- Carry your idea journal with you in a purse or pocket and have another near your bed at night so that it will be easily accessible when an inspiring idea comes along.

- Try timed brainstorming sessions by setting a timer for five minutes to list all the ideas you can think of for a particular subject matter (the plot for that book you always waned to write, must haves for the house you'd like to purchase one day, ways to become more fit, a themed social gathering you want to host, fundraising options for the nonprofit where you volunteer). There are no bad ideas at this stage so don't hold back.

- You may also wish to set a specific time to devote to creative thinking each day. Many people find early morning the perfect time to let their creativity flow. You may allot as much or as little time as you choose, but choose a time when you are sharp, relaxed, and undistracted.

Directions: Throughout this week endeavor to write in your creativity journal daily until it becomes a part of your routine. Use the following ideas to get started or generate your own.

1. Throughout your day think about which designs/products/processes you encounter that frustrate you most. Challenge yourself to create a better prototype.

2. Sit for a period of time in a place other than work or home such as a park, coffee shop, shopping mall, or airport (if you happen to be traveling). Record the stimuli you absorb – sights, sounds, smells, tastes, textures.

3. Design a new children's toy.

4. List unusual uses for a common household object such as a rubber band or coffee mug. Give yourself five minutes to develop a comprehensive list.

5. Try toppling, the concept of generating new words, from free association. If you chose the word ball, you might think of the word round, then the word globe, then the word plane, and so on.

6. Sometimes we have difficulty solving a problem because we aren't asking the right question. Try this exercise to help generate questions. Ask yourself a basic question. For example, how could I improve my health? Quickly, without overthinking, come up with 10 variations of the same question. What do I need to do to live an optimal life? What is my biggest obstacle to eating better? What is the best way to harness physical energy?

7. Compare two objects that do not appear similar on the surface. Think outside the box to determine properties they have in common.

8. Imagine yourself as someone very different from yourself – a dancer, senator, exchange student, stand up comedian, architect. How would your life be different? What characteristics of your personality would actually aide in that position?

9. Think of learning something you've never done before. Break down the steps of how you would master it.

10. Answer creative questions: What is my favorite vacation memory? What can I learn from young children? If I were the only survivor of a plane crash in the jungle, how would I survive? What career would I like to experience for a day? If I could construct the house of my dreams, what would it look like? What three things would I take with me to live on an island? What would my platform be if I was running for a political office?

ADDITIONAL NOTES:

_____

_____

_____

_____

+ EARTH

CONSERVATION

Earth provides enough to satisfy every man's needs, but not every man's greed.

— MAHATMA GANDHI

Background

The environmental movement in the United States began in the late 19th century, out of concern for the natural resources of the West. John Muir and Henry David Thoreau were key figures in the effort following Thoreau's reflective book *Walden*, espousing simple living in natural surroundings and the establishment of the Sierra Club by Muir in 1892. The decimation of the American Bison and death of the last passenger pigeon in the beginning of the 20th century helped popularize their concerns with the general population. President Roosevelt brought conservation into the political arena by setting aside land for national parks.

Getting Started

Without conscious awareness, many of our daily habits end up wasting needless energy. By making a few simple adjustments you can eliminate waste and help preserve our earth's resources. Things as simple as turning off your appliances while not in use and switching to energy efficient light bulbs help reduce carbon emission. Begin with three or four small changes, and once those become part of your normal routine, select three or four more.

Noteworthy

- *Think twice before you buy it*: In a society where consumption is at an all time high, it is easy to believe there is something new out there we must have. Resist the urge to turn over your material belongings continually by becoming a conscientious shopper. When you do purchase an item, make thoughtful choices that will last well into the future. When possible, donate or recycle the items you are replacing so that they don't end up in the landfill.

- *Live more simply*: Striving to live more simply will achieve the dual purpose of helping preserve the environment and decreasing daily stress. This includes being happier with what you already have and not allowing additional items to clutter your home, shopping locally when you do need to buy something, combining errands to save on gas consumption (or taking your bike), and eating whole food rather than processed.

- *Turn it down, turn it off*: Heating and cooling systems are tremendous energy hogs. Water and space heating account for nearly 63 percent of typical energy use. Install a programmable thermostat to reduce energy while you are away or sleeping. Turn down your water heater by a few degrees and your appliances off when not in use. Consider a home audit to uncover more ways to improve energy efficiency.

Directions: In the coming week strive to change your consumption habits with these simple suggestions:

Don't rinse: Stop rinsing plates before using your dishwasher and you save 20 gallons of water each load.

Use fewer napkins: The average American uses approximately 2,200 napkins a year, or six a day. If everyone used one less a day it would save more than a billion pounds from landfills annually.

Turn them off: Turn off computers in the evening rather than keeping in sleep mode to save 40 watts each day. Boot up while you making your coffee.

Stop paper bank statement: If every household took advantage of online bank statements, the money saved could send more than 17,000 high school graduates to a public university for a year.

Use rechargeable batteries: Each year 15 billion batteries are purchased and most are disposable alkaline batteries, with only a fraction being recycled.

Use paperboard spindle cotton swabs: If 10 percent of U.S. households switched from plastic to paperboard spindle swabs, the petroleum energy saved per year would be equivalent to over 150,000 gallons of gasoline.

Stop the answering machine: Answering machines use energy 24 hours each day and are put in landfills when they break. If everyone switched to an answering service, we would save nearly 2 billion kilowatt-hours.

Download your software: More than 30 billion compact discs are sold annually. Downloading your software has the added bonus of being available at a later date in the event you upgrade a computer.

Go to a professional car wash: Professional car washes are far more efficient with water consumption. If everyone in the U.S. who washed their car took just one trip to the car wash we could save nearly 8.7 billion gallons.

Choose matches over lighters: Most lighters are made out of plastic and filled with butane fluid, both petroleum products. Over 1.5 billion end up in landfills each year.

Keep fireplace damper closed: Leaving your fireplace damper open when not in use is akin to leaving a 48-inch window open during the winter.

Recycle old cell phones: The average cell phone lasts approximately 18 months, which means 130 million phones will be retired each year.

Invest in your own coffee cup: Investing in a reusable cup not only cuts down on waste, but keeps your coffee much hotter. Most coffee shops will happily fill your own cup, and may even give you a discount.

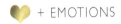

CARD OF APPRECIATION

Appreciation can make a day, even change a life. Your willingness to put it into words is all that is necessary.

— MARGARET COUSINS

Background

Expressing gratitude is a well-documented intentional activity that raises levels of happiness and well being. Beyond the generic gratitude lists we are all familiar with, cards of appreciation are a simple and inexpensive way to thank those who have made a difference in our life. Not only will the recipient be imbued with feelings of good will from the expression of your gratitude, but you as the writer will benefit from positive emotions as well. All that is required is a notecard, a recipient in mind, and a few moments of thoughtful reflection.

Getting Started

Make a habit of showing your appreciation for the various people in your life by sending a card of appreciation to a deserving individual at least once a month. Recipients might include family members who have contributed to your welfare over the years, close friends who always have been supportive, a professional who has gone above and beyond in terms of services rendered, neighbors who have been particularly kind, a co-worker who helped you out of a sticky situation, or someone you simply feel would benefit from an extra kind word.

Noteworthy

- Be on the lookout for unique and beautiful cards at specialty stores such as museum gift shops and fine stationers. Or, increase the enjoyment of this task by creating your own card using the wealth of scrapbooking supplies available at most craft stores.

- Be sure to include in your card the specific behavior you are appreciative of, the impact it has had on your life, and an acknowledgment of the time and effort on the part of the recipient.

- Sometimes we put off such cards of appreciation and gratitude because we fear being clumsy in our wording or not being able to find the right words. Keep the cards manageable in terms of length and complexity. It is so rare these days to receive an actual hand-written note that the recipient is bound to be delighted with the special recognition regardless what is said on the card itself.

Directions: Begin the practice of sending a card of appreciation monthly to someone who inspires gratitude in you due to their kindness or support.

POSSIBLE RECIPIENTS:

MONTHLY CARDS:

JANUARY |

FEBRUARY |

MARCH |

APRIL |

MAY |

JUNE |

JULY |

AUGUST |

SEPTEMBER |

OCTOBER |

NOVEMBER |

DECEMBER |

ADDITIONAL NOTES:

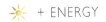

ENERGY BOOSTERS

The groundwork of all happiness is health.

— LEIGH HUNT

Background

The touchstone of good health should first and foremost be adequate energy for the myriad of tasks we are called upon to complete within a typical day. Major factors that contribute to decreased energy include unhealthy diets, inadequate sleep, too much stress, and not enough exercise. But sometimes energy zappers come in less obvious forms such as too much time on our electronic devices, caring for young children or aging parents, too much caffeine, and an excessive amount of sitting at work or home. The result is gradually depleted energy stores that leave us sluggish, irritable, and unable to concentrate.

Getting Started

Once the larger issues of diet, sleep, and exercise are considered, begin refining your energy habits still further until you regularly experience abundant energy from the time you awake until you retire to bed in the evening. Many of the suggestions found on the following page are common-sense solutions that oftentimes get overlooked. Although the individual benefit may be subtle, they are all positive conduits for energy. Keeping track of your efforts and the effect on overall energy by means of a journal or app will allow you to develop a positive mind-body connection of healthy habits you are more likely to maintain.

Noteworthy

* Our thoughts are another source of energy, both positive and negative. If you spend time ruminating about past mistakes, angrily recalling an irritating situation, or wishing you'd been given different life circumstances, you run the risk of interfering with endorphins that promote health, relaxation, and vibrant energy.

* Along the same lines, be careful about overly ambitious goal setting and the elusive pursuit of perfectionism. Psychologists have found elevated levels of Creactive protein, an indicator of inflammation, in people who were unable to relinquish unobtainable goals. This sort of *all or nothing* thinking creates more than just negative energy; it sets the stage for the possibility of genuine illness.

* Laughing and socially connecting with others are two excellent ways to keep your energy level high due to the positive mental and physical benefits of both. Plan regular social opportunities throughout your week and enhance the benefit by attending a comedy club or having a game night.

Directions: Try these energy boosters throughout your week to help combat midday slumps.

Head outside: Sunlight has the profound ability to energize you and elevate your mood. Try to spend a few minutes outside each day, away from the dulling effect of fluorescent lighting and computer screens. If it's warm enough to slip off your shoes, you'll experience even greater energy with your feet actually in grass. The act of allowing your skin to come into contact with the earth is called grounding or earthing.

Finish your shower with cold water: Use the last 2–3 minutes of your morning shower to get a quick pick-me-up by turning the temperature fairly chilly. You instantly will notice the stimulating effect of this simple exercise. Splashing cool water on your face after a vigorous workout will accomplish the same thing.

Eat smaller meals more frequently: Rather than three large meals, which can make you sleepy as your body works to digest the food, try smaller amounts more frequently throughout the day. This will provide a steady stream of nutrients to your mind and body. This is particularly true at lunch. Researchers have found people who have a big lunch typically experience an afternoon slump.

Listen to music: The reason we exercise to music is because music is extremely motivating and energizing, especially if you sing along. Researchers in London found that singing solo increases physical energy and decreases tension almost as much as a cardio workout. If you get up to listen to the music, that's even better. The simple act of standing provides an instant energy surge.

Switch to tea: Rather than your usual cup of coffee, try swapping for a cup of green tea instead. Green tea not only has smaller amounts of caffeine, but contains the active compound EGCG, which facilitates weight loss. Green tea in the afternoon is also less likely to interfere with your sleep schedule.

Pop a piece of gum: A 2012 study from the UK concluded that chewing gum for 15 minutes increases alertness by increasing heart rate, which increases blood flow to the brain. It also stimulates the autonomic nervous system, which increases alertness. Choose mint for the greatest effect.

Eat complex carbs and less sugar: Studies have shown glucose from complex carbs like whole grains make subjects feels more energized. Decreasing sugar will keep blood sugar balanced by avoiding the immediate spike that comes with eating something sweet, followed by the rapid drop in blood sugar, which can leave you feeling sluggish.

Sit up straight: Slouching over a computer for long periods can cause fatigue during the day. By sitting up straight with your shoulders back, eyes ahead, and lower back slightly arched you will instantly feel more alert and strong. If you switch gears once you start feeling sleepy and engage in something new and interesting, you can beat back a lack of energy still further. The more actively you engage your brain, the more alert you will feel.

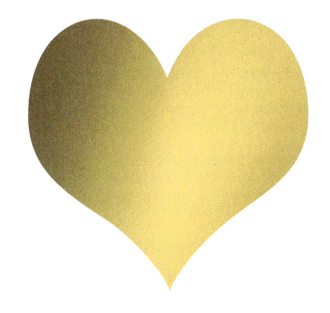

+ EMOTION

(AUTHENTIC HAPPINESS)

Raise your happiness level by increasing the occurrence of positive emotions through the science of happiness

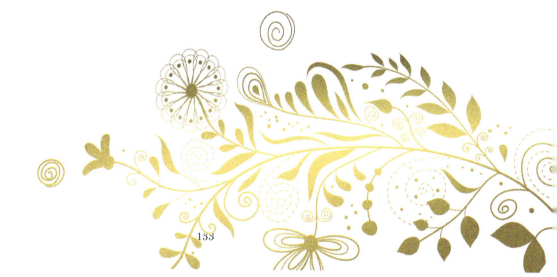

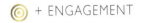

MONTHLY CULTURAL GOAL

Man's mind, once stretched by a new idea, never regains its original dimensions.
— OLIVER WENDELL HOLMES

Background

A substantial study by Koenraad Cuypers involving 50,797 Norwegians found that participation in cultural events was significantly associated with robust health, greater satisfaction with life, and lowered rates of anxiety and depression in both genders. Not only do we benefit mentally from quality cultural experiences, but we also gain the additional benefits of connecting with others socially and altruistically when we help support the cultural nonprofit organizations within our communities. In a 2007 commencement address at Stanford University, poet and chairman for the National Endowment of the Arts, Dana Giola stated, "Art is an irreplaceable way of understanding and expressing the world. There are some truths about life that can be expressed only as stories, or songs, or images. Art delights, instructs, consoles. It educates our emotions."

Getting Started

If you have a tendency to confine yourself to the familiar comfort of your home rather than venturing out for an evening of culture, set a monthly goal that will encourage you to try something new in the coming year. Begin by scouring the entertainment section of the newspaper or going online to your community calendar to access upcoming cultural events that fit within your personal schedule and budget. If you have difficulty enticing your spouse for such an endeavor, contact one or more close friends and organize a monthly evening on the town.

Noteworthy

- To expand your cultural experience further research the composer, playwright, artist, musical piece, art installation, historical era or speaker prior to the event and/or journal your impressions afterwards.

- Most communities offer multiple museums, art galleries, theater settings, and historical sites, which can be rotated to maximize the potential for a variety of experiences.

- If you would like to attempt an even more ambitious goal, strive to see a live performance monthly in addition to visiting a museum, art gallery, or historical site.

- Don't forget to include evidence of your monthly cultural goal (i.e. playbills, ticket stubs, programs, and informational flyers) to your Learning Inspiration Board.

Directions: Complete the form each month upon reaching your cultural goal.

JANUARY	MONTHLY CULTURAL GOAL:
DATE COMPLETED:

FEBRUARY	MONTHLY CULTURAL GOAL:
DATE COMPLETED:

MARCH	MONTHLY CULTURAL GOAL:
DATE COMPLETED:

APRIL	MONTHLY CULTURAL GOAL:
DATE COMPLETED:

MAY	MONTHLY CULTURAL GOAL:
DATE COMPLETED:

JUNE	MONTHLY CULTURAL GOAL:
DATE COMPLETED:

JULY	MONTHLY CULTURAL GOAL:
DATE COMPLETED:

AUGUST	MONTHLY CULTURAL GOAL:
DATE COMPLETED:

SEPTEMBER	MONTHLY CULTURAL GOAL:
DATE COMPLETED:

OCTOBER	MONTHLY CULTURAL GOAL:
DATE COMPLETED:

NOVEMBER	MONTHLY CULTURAL GOAL:
DATE COMPLETED:

DECEMBER	MONTHLY CULTURAL GOAL:
DATE COMPLETED:

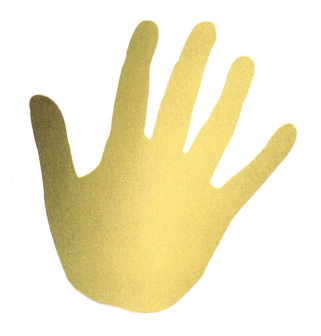

+ ENCOUNTERS

(SOCIAL CONNECTIONS)

Celebrate the power of friendship,
the perfect antidote for successful aging

GAME NIGHT

Never, ever underestimate the importance of having fun.

— RANDY PAUSCH

Background

Board games date back as early as 2500 B.C. with nearly every culture and society throughout history able to boast of such organized entertainment in some form, although it wasn't until much later that they gained in widespread popularity. As the United States shifted from agrarian to urban living in the 19th century, greater leisure time and a rise in income became available to the middle class. The American home became the heart of entertainment, enlightenment, and education within the family. Children were encouraged to play board games that developed literacy skills and promoted moral instruction.

Getting Started

Play is a concept that shouldn't be limited to children, as it is equally as important in the lives of adults. Scheduled play in the form of game nights can be an inviting source of relaxation and stimulation that benefits all parties involved. Strive to set aside one evening a month for playing board games with family members or friends. Playing regularly has the potential to bring increased joy, vitality, and resilience to your relationships, simultaneously healing minor disagreements and resentments that arise from time to time.

Noteworthy

- One of the best benefits of playing games is the hilarity that such evenings provide. It is difficult to play any board game for long without regular doses of laughter, all of which positively affect the participants. Laughter relaxes the entire body, boosts the immune system, protects the heart, and increases the release of endorphins, the body's natural feel-good chemicals.

- Social connections and laughter aren't the only positive outcomes from playing board games. If you choose games that require problem solving and criticalthinking skills, there is a mental benefit as well, which aids in staving off later-life dementia.

- Playing games keeps us young and energetic, even going so far as to improve our resistance to disease. In the words of George Bernard Shaw, "We don't stop playing because we grow old; we grow old because we stop playing."

Directions: Enjoy a game night with friends or family using the following suggestions.

Guest List: Keep the guest list to 12 or fewer so that logistical details don't become overwhelming. Strive for a variety of personalities, which will make the evening more entertaining. This is a good opportunity to "mix" your usual groups so that guests get a chance to meet others in a relaxed atmosphere.

Invitations: When inviting people for the first time to an evening of games, explain in detail the purpose of the get together, focusing on the social aspect of the evening. Many individuals harbor negative associations of games due to previous experiences that have resulted in boredom or embarrassment. Let your guests know that a few games will be played with directions given.

Food: Game nights are perfect opportunities for a potluck with the host being responsible for the main course and guests bringing side dishes. Have a few snacks available upon arrival with the remainder of the meal served later in the evening. Due to the fun nature of the activity, you may choose to have guests come earlier than they normally would with a couple games played before eating. During game playing, have a side table available for food and drinks to avoid spills onto the board.

Directions: Be considerate of those guests who do not have a great deal of game playing experience by thoroughly explaining rules and allowing a practice round before the competition begins. Strive to choose games that would appeal to a large range of people without embarrassing anyone (although part of the appeal of games is the ridiculous situations people find themselves and their ability to laugh at the situation).

Variety of Games: Card games are an easy, inexpensive way to begin a game night, particularly if you have invited 2–3 couples, since many games are played in partnership. Options include hearts, spades, pitch, 500, and canasta. In addition, there are numerous board games that will appeal to a wide array of players and are engaging as well. Top rated board games include: Ticket to Ride, Scrabble, Risk, Apples to Apples, Clue, Yahtzee, Trivial Pursuit, Pictionary, Taboo, Uno, and Scattergories.

ADDITIONAL NOTES FOR YOUR GAME NIGHT:

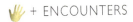

HOST YOUR OWN OKTOBERFEST

Fall has always been my favorite season. The time when everything bursts with its last beauty, as if nature has been saving up all year for the grand finale.

— LAUREN DESTEFANO

Background

Oktoberfest, generally accepted as the world's largest fair, is held annually in the Bavarian region of Munich, Germany. This sixteen-day festival runs from late September to the first weekend of October and attracts some six million people from around the world. Revelers are treated to traditional German music while they feast on roast chicken, pork, ham hock, bratwurst, pretzels, potato dumplings, red cabbage, and, of course, beer. Today, cities and towns around Germany and across the world celebrate their own versions of Oktoberfest, modeled after the Munich event.

Getting Started

Autumn is an ideal season for entertaining due to its pleasant temperatures, colorful backdrop, and un-official end of summer holidays. Consider gathering a group together to celebrate autumn with your own personalized Oktoberfest celebration. This special social event could be planned for family members, close friends, or surrounding neighbors. Nearly everyone is thrilled by an invitation to spend an evening in the company of others. When a fun and unique theme is involved, you're guaranteed guests won't want to miss the occasion.

Noteworthy

- Only beer brewed that meets strict requirements and is brewed within Munich city limits qualifies to be served at Oktoberfest. The higher alcohol content of Oktoberfest beer (5.8 – 6.3 percent) along with high sugar content, frequently causes many people to overestimate their ability to handle the alcohol. Drunken patrons are referred to as *bierleichen* ("beer corpses") by the German.

- Oktoberfest of 2010 marked the two-hundred year anniversary of the event, which originated as a wedding celebration of Crown Prince Ludwig to Princess Therese of Saxe – Hildburghausen. It was from the bride's moniker that the fields where the festivities took place were named *Theresienwiese*. The locals later abbreviated this to simply *Wiesn*.

- The first carousel to be set up at an Oktoberfest arrived in 1818. Today carousels, roller coasters, and other fun activities for people of all ages are available at the foot of the Bavaria Statue, adjacent to festival grounds.

Directions: Consider the following suggestions when hosting your own Oktoberfest celebration:

O **Onset**: Once you have set a date, invite friends to your event, making sure your invitations keep with the fall theme.

K **Keep in simple**: The most successful entertainers understand the importance of keeping things simple. Don't become overwhelmed by making the party overly complicated or stressful. If you are at ease, your guests will be as well.

T **Table**: Make the table where folks will be eating the focal point with autumn colored placemats or table-cloth, pots of mums or other fall flowers, and leaves and gourds scattered across the top.

O **Outside or in**: If the weather where you live is fairly predictable, move the party outdoors if possible. You might even choose to erect a small tent to convey the spirit of the festival. Renovated garages are another possibility that provide an outdoor feel while still being covered in the event of inclement weather.

B **Beer**: Highlight the featured alcohol by having a wide variety of beers or having guests bring different types for all to sample. You will want to provide a limited selection of wine as well for non-beer drinkers.

E **Entertainment**: Add another level of festivity to the evening with traditional German music. The lively sounds of an oompah band playing in the background is guaranteed to keep everyone in high spirits.

R **Recruit**: You will find yourself frazzled by the end of the evening unless you elicit the help of others. Ask various friends to help refresh drinks, attend to music, take pictures, or stack dirty dishes in the kitchen.

F **Food**: Oktoberfest food is fairly simple and hearty. Grilled brats, potato salad and red cabbage slaw are the perfect food fare here. If you have access to an antique milk can, consider a Milk Can Dinner where sausages, potatoes, corn on the cob, and cabbage are layered into the can and steamed to smoky perfection.

E **Exult in the season**: Make the most of the lingering warm days by adorning your house inside and out with evidence of fall's splendor.

S **Send off**: Send your guests home with a reminder of the fun evening by providing them with homemade caramel apples or pecan pralines as they leave.

T **Tradition**: Consider making your Oktoberfest an annual tradition, anticipated by all who attended the previous year.

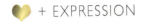

OVERCOMING CREATIVITY ROADBLOCKS

Every child is an artist, the problem is staying an artist when you grow up.

— PABLO PICASSO

Background

When Robert Fulgham wrote the poem All I Really Need to Know I Learned in Kindergarten, he might just as well have been referring to creativity. As humans, we are each born with an innate ability to be creative. Young children draw whatever pops into their heads and sing with abandon, they perform skits with or without an audience and invent silly games to pass the time — all without consideration for the end product, but for the sheer delight of doing so. One of the truly great tragedies of growing up is the inevitable loss of such uninhibited creativity, the gradual realization that perhaps we shouldn't be so casual with our creative efforts. For many of us, we close ourselves off to future creative endeavors.

Getting Started

It is as important to be aware of those things we do that impede creativity as those that foster it. This begins with negative self-talk that tries to convince us some people are creative and others are not. Once you come to understand creativity better, you will discover it is not a question of whether creativity is inherent in you — it is inherent in all of us — but rather how often you will allow yourself time to explore this dimension. In the coming week, challenge yourself to look at whatever obstacles or roadblocks to creativity you might be encountering on a daily basis and consider ways to overcome them.

Noteworthy

- Creativity helps us to live in the present moment, to see things from different angles and to brainstorm and problem solve, all of which help serve you when facing difficult life decisions or situations.

- Being creative is not a passive process, subsequently creative people are more responsive to sensory stimulation. In addition, they have higher baseline levels of arousal and increased goal-directed behavior. (Psychology Today, 2010)

- Nearly 75 percent of people believe they are not living up to their creative potential. One of the biggest roadblocks is the simple pattern of human habit. Once we start doing something one way, we get overly comfortable and are not prone to change.

Directions: Most of our obstacles to creativity lie within us. Check to make sure your creative efforts are not suffering from the following obstacles:

Fear

Fear is perhaps the most challenging obstacle to overcome due to its ubiquitous presence in the creative process. The success of any creative endeavor is unknown and, therefore, unsettling. We fear criticism (our own and others), time and/or money wasted, and an inability to capture what we are hoping to portray. Overcoming our own self-doubt is the first step in allowing creativity to occur.

Create positive affirmations that will buoy you when you find yourself lacking confidence in a creative endeavor. Post them so they are visible when you work.

Perfectionism

Everyone wants to do well when they attempt something, but seeking perfection almost always gets in the way of creative pursuits. By worrying too much about how something will "turn out," we pour energy into the end result rather than the process. If we force our project into a preconceived notion of how it should look, we don't allow the creativity to take over in an organic way.

While it is important to have direction and plan out your project, resist the urge to focus on a set end product. Allow your unconscious self to flow with the activity in whatever way it chooses.

Lack of Vision

Often people think too narrowly when considering what they can accomplish. Because of this they stay within their comfort zone when it comes to the creative process, failing to use their imagination about possibilities. On the other end of the spectrum are those who think too broadly when it comes to planning their projects without time line or plan of action.

Challenge yourself to try something you've never attempted before, making sure you are clear on what you want to accomplish and how you will get there.

Environment

This may seem obvious, but an appropriate setting for your creative work is essential. A space that is too sterile, cluttered, noisy, or uninviting is bound to have a stifling effect on your work. Seriously consider where you are most likely to accomplish your creative goals. It should be convenient for storing necessary tools and away from most interruptions.

Make a list of what you most need in your environment to be successful and set about making it happen; research solutions for small spaces if appropriate.

ADDITIONAL NOTES:

CHRISTMAS CHEER

Somehow, not only for Christmas, but all the long year through, the joy that you give to others, is the joy that comes back to you.

— JOHN GREENLEAF WHITTIER

Background

There's something about Christmas that encourages us to look beyond ourselves to the needs of our fellow man, those individuals without the basic necessities we often take for granted. Perhaps it is the realization that we are all generally more blessed than we, at times, acknowledge. This season, consider the particular skills and talents you might contribute to an organization and then find time between your social activities to give back to the less fortunate citizens within your community. You will most assuredly be rewarded with a gift too expansive to fit in a box.

Getting Started

Don't wait until the last moment to get involved with community opportunities, as they tend to fill up quickly. Some shelters and soup kitchens report filling volunteer slots a year in advance. Keep an eye out for posters, newspaper ads, or bulletin board notices at your local library, grocery store, and mall. Whether or not you belong to a church, most would welcome the efforts of non-members. Internet searches are guaranteed to present numerous opportunities as well. Begin by considering your time, energy, skills, and resources when determining where you are a good fit.

Noteworthy

- If your experience volunteering during the holiday season is a positive one, consider continuing throughout the coming year. Many organizations are well aware of citizens wanting to help at Christmas time, but desperately need the help every month.

- Spreading Christmas cheer to those less fortunate is the perfect antidote to the requisite gluttony that accompanies a holiday season filled with excessive eating, drinking, materialism, and festivity. If this time of year tends to make you anxious or depressed, concentrating on those who are marginalized by circumstances will shift your focus in a positive direction.

- If children have a special place in your heart, consider such organizations as Angel Tree (gifts for children of prisoners), Operation Christmas Child (shoeboxes filled with supplies for children), Make-a-Wish Foundation (for terminally ill children), Toys For Tots, and My Two Front Teeth (personalized gift giving to aid underprivileged children).

Directions: Identify the right volunteering opportunity for your community and make the call.

- If you have musical talent such as playing the guitar or piano, consider performing Christmas carols at a nursing home or assisted care facility.

- Because of a spike of violence at Christmas time, most women and children shelters are in need of extra donations including clothing, toiletries, and diapers. If you enjoy working with kids, consider supervising a craft activity with the children at a shelter.

- The staff of an animal shelter would gladly welcome extra help walking boarded animals, particularly on Christmas Eve or Christmas Day.

- Many churches and organizations offer programs to adopt a low-income family, providing them Christmas dinner and gifts.

- Likewise, most major shopping centers provide trees with gift requests that you can sponsor. These include not only children, but teens, and seniors as well. Choose a group closest to your heart.

- Reliable organizations such as Salvation Army and United Way are sure to have opportunities available throughout the holiday season. Local food pantries will be in need of individuals to assemble and distribute food boxes.

- Call your local United Service Organization, Veterans of Foreign Wars, Veterans Administration hospital and other veteran organizations to find out whether they have any need for volunteers this holiday season.

- Contact your local hospital and ask whether you could make get well cards for children in the pediatric unit. Spend a day with friends making them and drop them off for distribution.

- A simple way to spread Christmas cheer is by providing baked goods for those under recognized individuals who serve the community including police, fire fighters, animal shelter staff, and social workers.

NOTES:

_____

_____

_____

_____

_____

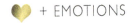 + EMOTIONS

BEST-SELF LIFE

You only live once, but if you do it right, once is enough.

— MAE WEST

Background

Visualization has been popular since the Soviets began using it in the 1970s for sports competitions. Brain studies now reveal thoughts produce the exact same mental instructions as actions and mental practices are nearly as effective as actual physical activity. Mental imagery impacts a number of cognitive processes in the brain including motor control, attention, perception, planning, and memory. In addition, it's been found that mental practice enhances motivation, increases confidence and self-efficacy, improves motor performance, primes your brain for success, and increases states of flow. In this strategy you will begin using the powerful practice of visualization to help create your best possible life.

Getting Started

The first step to achieving the life we want is to have a clear image of what that looks like specifically. This week begin considering every detail of your perfect life from what home you'd like to reside in to what adventures you'd like to pursue. Keep in mind this blueprint for the future should be genuine to you and not based on any cultural stereotypes of the "good life." For many, living in a cozy cottage would be much preferable to a rambling estate. Once you finish formulating a description for the different categories of your richly imagined life, hold a mental image as if it were happening at this moment using all five of your senses. Revisit your ideal future on a regular basis, editing the information accordingly.

Noteworthy

- Mental imagery studies reveal the strength of the mind-body connection, the link between your thoughts and behavior. This is an extremely important connection for achieving your best life.

- Visualization of goals and desires accomplishes three things: 1) it activates your creative subconscious, which will start generating creative ideas to achieve your goal; 2) it programs your brain to perceive and recognize more readily the resources needed to accomplish your goal; 3) it builds your internal motivation to take the necessary steps to achieve your dream.

- It may take some time to feel comfortable with visualization of your best life, so be patient with the process. The more detail you can provide to your picture, the more likely you are to achieve it.

Directions: At least once a year, devote genuine time and effort to visualizing your Best-Self Life. Begin by filling in your ideal vision for each of the following categories.

BEST-SELF LIFE INVENTORY

Personal skills you'd like to acquire:

_____

_____

_____

_____

_____

Passions you'd like to explore:

_____

_____

_____

_____

_____

Places you'd like to travel:

_____

_____

_____

_____

_____

Environment you'd like to create:

_____

_____

_____

_____

_____

BEST-SELF LIFE INVENTORY

Social connections you'd like to establish:

_____
_____
_____
_____

Adventures you'd like to have:

_____
_____
_____
_____

Items you'd like to possess:

_____
_____
_____
_____

Family you'd like to nurture:

_____
_____
_____
_____

Careers you'd like to pursue:

_____
_____
_____
_____

Accomplishments you'd like to achieve:

_____
_____
_____
_____

ADDITIONAL NOTES:

BOXING DAY

May no gift be too small to give, nor too simple to receive, which is wrapped in thoughtfulness and tied with love.

— LAUREN DESTEFANO

Background

The European tradition called Boxing Day began in England in the Middle Ages when servants were required to work on Christmas, but had the following day (December 26th) off. With all the servants gathered together at one time, the lords of the manors would present them with gift boxes filled with food and other necessities that were due them for the coming year. As time went by, the tradition spread to those who had rendered a service during the year and became voluntary in nature rather than required by the employer. Today, the tradition survives as people give presents to tradesmen, mail carriers, porters, and others to express their gratitude.

Getting Started

We all have individuals in our personal circles that make life easier thanks to the services they provide. These might include the barista at our favorite coffee house, our salon stylist, the gym class instructor, our paper and mail carrier, the individual who dry cleans our clothes, our dog sitter, and countless others. Let them know how much they are appreciated by devoting a day each year to recognize them. This can either be done on December 26th in keeping with the Boxing Day spirit, or at a less busy time of year. All that is required is a simple token of appreciation (multiplied by the number of individuals you are gifting) and a pretty bag or small box.

Noteworthy

- For many countries Boxing Day is a bank holiday observed most notably in European countries, but also in Canada, Hong Kong, Australia and New Zealand; Kenya, South Africa, and Guyana; as well as the Scandinavia countries. In South Africa, the day is known as the Day of Goodwill, while in Ireland, Italy, Finland, and parts of France, the day is known as St. Stephen's Day.

- A second version of how Boxing Day may have originated is attributed to the Church of England. It seems during Advent, Anglican parishes displayed a box for monetary donations to be made by church-goers. On the day after Christmas, the boxes were broken open and their contents distributed among the poor.

- Today, Boxing Day is primarily a day to relax with football matches, horse racing, and shopping among the activities favored.

Directions: Use the following ideas for your Boxing Day gifts. Place in a stylish container, such as decorative boxes or pretty fabric bags, which can be found at any craft store.

Homemade goodies such as salsa, jam, biscotti, or candy

Paper products such as notecards and stamps, entertaining plates and napkins, or notepads and pens

Specialty chocolate such as Godiva or Ghirardelli

Bath products such as lotion, bath oil, scrubbing salts, or hand cream

Gift cards to restaurants or stores

Items from Christmas craft fairs such as scarves, mittens, jewelry, or candles

ADDITIONAL BOXING DAY IDEAS:

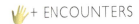 + ENCOUNTERS

LIGHT YOUR WAY TO THE NEW YEAR

Ring out the old, ring in the new, Ring, happy bells, across the snow: The year is going, let it go; Ring out the false, ring in the true.

— ALFRED, LORD TENNYSON

Background

We are all looking for meaningful ways to ring in the New Year and sharing your own version of *Loy Krathong* with friends and family may be just the answer. *Loy Krathong* is a visually spectacular Thai festival held on the full moon of the twelfth month in the traditional Thai lunar calendar. *Loi* means "to float" and *krathong* refers to a tiny raft traditionally made from a section of banana tree trunk, decorated with elaborately-folded banana leaves, flowers, candles, incense sticks, etc. During the night of the full moon, people release these small rafts onto the river, believing that floating a krathong will create good luck. Loy Krathong coincides with the Lanna festival in northern Thailand known as *Yi Peng*. During Yi Peng a multitude of Lanna-style sky lanterns (*khom fai*) are launched into the skies where they resemble large flocks of giant fluorescent jellyfish gracefully floating overhead.

Getting Started

Instead of the ubiquitous drinks, appetizers, and small talk that accompany most New Year's Eve parties, why not consider bringing close friends together for an end-of-the year celebration centered around the beautiful ritual of Loy Krathong. This activity calls for an area away from food and drink to construct each "raft," a small assortment of supplies, and a vessel with which to display the works of art. At the end of the evening the small homemade boat serves as a favor, reminding them of their hopes for the New Year.

Noteworthy

- The Loy Krathong festival originated in Thailand to honor Buddha. The candle exalts the Buddha with light, while the floating krathong symbolizes letting go of one's hatred, anger, and defilements. Thai natives sometimes place fingernail or hair clippings on the krathong as a symbol of letting go of negative thoughts.

- In the opening scenes of the 2012 movie *The Impossible*, which captured the devastating 2004 Indian Ocean tsunami as experienced by Maria Belon and her family, there is a lanna lighting ceremony of sky lanterns that showcases the unique beauty of this ritual.

- Biodegradable sky lanterns can also be purchased online through a variety of websites.

Directions: Use the following steps to help bring a bit of Thai to your next New Year's Eve party.

Supplies: You will need to purchase tea lights, very small plastic containers (such as to hold condiments), colored Sharpies to decorate the containers, and fresh flowers (optional). Another option if you can find them, is to purchase floating candles in the shape of flowers and use a small wooden skewer pushed into the wax with a paper banner taped to the top of the skewer for guests to decorate.

Upon arrival: Once guests arrive, have them select a tea light, plastic container, and Sharpie. On the bottom of the tea light they are to write one negative thing they wish to say good-bye to from the past year. On the container itself, they should write one hope for the coming year. They can finish their project by adding a small fresh flower to the container.

Display: To display the decorated rafts you will need to have a large vessel available to float them upon. Any type of large bowl with a wide surface area would work. This should be placed in an area of the room that is visible to partygoers, but dimly lit to showcase the candles. If you have a small kiddie pool, this could even be done on a patio close to glass sliding doors.

Departing: Don't forget to allow each guest to take home his or her container as a memento of the evening. The tea candles with outgoing regrets can be tossed and the container with inspirational message and fresh flowers presented as a keepsake.

Other considerations: If purchasing sky lanterns to release at some point during the evening rather than creating rafts to float, messages can be written onto paper and tied to lanterns beforehand. To keep with the ambience of the party, consider serving Thai food that is either purchased from a local restaurant, homemade if you enjoy cooking, or used as a potluck theme.

ADDITIONAL NOTES FOR YOUR EVENT:

ADDITIONAL NOTES:

ADDITIONAL NOTES:

ADDITIONAL NOTES:

Conclusion

Congratulations on completing the *Expanded Joy* program! It is my sincere hope you were able to give most of the various projects in the book a try and found their cumulative impact on your daily life to be beneficial. As you consider maintaining the program long term, there are a few considerations to bear in mind.

Now that you are familiar with the program projects, you will need to determine which strategies to incorporate into some form of regular practice. There are a number of variables that will affect this decision. The amount of time you have available due to a job, caring for children/grandchildren, or volunteer activities will naturally influence the number of strategies you are able to take on in the future. There are other considerations such as age, health, and resources that may play a role in how many strategies you are able to undertake.

Start small by choosing one or two activities to maintain daily, weekly, or monthly. Keep track of their impact on your life and as time goes along determine whether you wish to continue them or discard accordingly. Once you are comfortable with these strategies, choose one or two more, weighing the benefits of each until you have created a program of joy that fits your needs. One thing to remember is that utilizing the strategies is like taking medicine, most are effective only while actively working them. Their effect fades fairly quickly upon cessation.

As mentioned in the Introduction, the *Expanded Joy* program is perhaps most effective when carried out with a partner or in a small group. The support and encouragement of others motivates us in ways we are sometimes unable to achieve otherwise. Just as you are more likely to go for that early morning walk when accompanied by a friend, you are also more likely to send off that Card of Appreciation or collect mementoes for your Laughter Treasure Trove when required to report back to others.

Above all, remember that the quest for joy is one that is ongoing. It doesn't matter where you are at on the joy continuum, only that you are moving forward on that continuum. Strive to make joyful living a priority this year, next year, and every year. It is the worthiest of goals, impacting not only your life, but the lives of all you encounter.

Acknowledgments

First and foremost, I would like to thank my husband, Steven Popish, for allowing me the luxury of this quest for joy that would not have been possible without his selfless support. And to my most precious daughters, Lauren and Julia, who have endured my all-consuming projects without complaint their entire lives. I also am deeply appreciative of those women whose friendships have played such a key role in my life. The women who, throughout the years, have shaped my existence, providing humor and strength, wisdom and serenity, all the necessary ingredients for joyful living.

I am forever indebted to the men and women who have made it their life work to research the areas of optimal living embraced within this book so that others might benefit. Individuals who have spent the bulk of their careers mapping out the specific components needed to live healthier, happier, more productively, and with greater resiliency. We have available today a body of information in the areas of health and wellness, positive psychology, neuroplasticity, flow, creativity, and philanthropy that is unprecedented in history. My work in trying to connect the research to the reader in a meaningful way was miniscule in comparison.

Above all, I would like to thank the stellar team of Elevate Publishing, particularly Mark Russell who initially saw promise in the concept. A special thanks to my perfect editor, Anna McHargue, whose incredible skills are eclipsed only by her flawless taste, as well as the invaluable assistance of Dave Troesh. And finally, to Bobby Kubler, who did a phenomenal job designing a beautiful book and then making it happen.

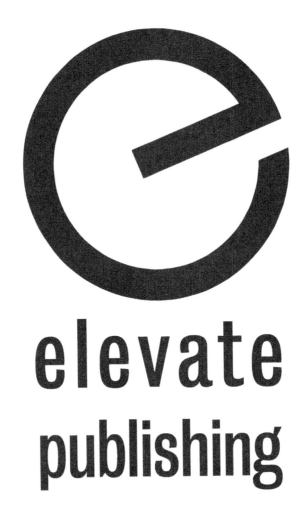

A strategic publisher empowering authors to strengthen their brand.

Visit Elevate Publishing for our latest offerings.
www.elevatepub.com

CPSIA information can be obtained at www.ICGtesting.com
Printed in the USA
BVOW10s1657111015

421774BV00005B/51/P

9 781937 498825